Common Gynecological Terms/Abbreviations

Term/Abbreviation	Definition
Adjuvant therapy	Complementary cancer treatment intended to impede the growth of micrometastatic disease
Amenorrhea (primary)	Absence of menarche by age 16 or absence of secondary sexual characteristics by age 14
Amenorrhea (secondary)	Absence of menses after history of established menstruation
Cervical dysplasia	Abnormal cervical cellular changes
Climacteric	Decline in female reproductive ability before menopause
Colporrhaphy	Surgical repair of weakened vaginal wall; used for treatment of rectocele (posterior)/cystocele (anterior)
Colposcope	Magnifying instrument used to closely examine cervical tissue and aid in biopsy if indicated
Corpus luteum	Term given to the follicle after ovulation; produces estrogen and progesterone in luteal phase of the menstrual cycle
Cryosurgery	Application of extremely cold cervical probe to the cervix intended to destroy and treat abnormal cervical cells
Cystocele	Protrusion of the bladder into the vagina
Dysmenorrhea	Painful menstruation
Dyspareunia	Pain experienced during intercourse
Endometriosis	Endometrial tissue located outside of the uterus
GnRH	Gona...
HPV	Hum...
Hysterectomy	Surg...
Hysterosalpingography	Radi... fall... me...

D0145911

Common Gynecological Terms/Abbreviations—cont'd

Term/Abbreviation	Definition
Hysteroscopy	Examination of the uterus using a specialized instrument
Kegel exercises	Exercises performed by a woman to strengthen the pelvic floor and decrease incidence of stress incontinence
LEEP	Loop electrosurgical excision procedure; used in the treatment of cervical dysplasia
Lymphedema	Abnormal accumulation of lymph fluid in the interstitial spaces; may occur after excision of lymph nodes
Mastectomy	Surgical removal of the breast
Menarche	Launch of menses in the young female
Menopause	Permanent cessation of menses marking the end of reproductive ability; average age in U.S. women, 52 years
Menorrhagia	Menstrual flow that is excessive in amount or number of days
Metrorrhagia	Bleeding between expected menstrual periods
Myomectomy	Surgical excision of a uterine fibroid
OC	Oral contraceptive
OCP	Oral contraceptive pill
Oligomenorrhea	Scanty or infrequent menstrual flow
Oophorectomy	Surgical excision of the ovary
Ovulation	Cyclic release of an ovum from graafian follicle; occurs 14 days before menses
PCOS	**P**olycystic **o**varian **s**yndrome
Pessary	Medical device used to support the pelvic floor and reduce symptoms associated with uterine prolapse, cystocele, and rectocele
Rectocele	Protrusion of the rectum into the vagina

Common Gynecological Terms/Abbreviations—cont'd

Term/Abbreviation	Definition
Salpingectomy	Surgical excision of the fallopian tube
Sentinel node	First lymph node that receives lymphatic drainage from a tumor
STD	**S**exually **t**ransmitted **d**isease
STI	**S**exually **t**ransmitted **i**nfection
TAH-BSO	**T**otal **a**bdominal **h**ysterectomy with **b**ilateral **s**alpingo-**o**ophorectomy
Uterine artery embolization	Procedure performed to decrease the blood supply to uterine fibroids, with the intention of shrinking them
Uterine fibroid	Encapsulated, connective tissue tumor of the uterus
Uterine prolapse	Protrusion of the uterus into the vagina

Ways That Nurses Have an Impact on Women's Health

Nurses have an impact on women's health through the following:
- Educating women about healthy lifestyle choices
- Role-modeling healthy behavior and promoting wellness
- Describing the role of prevention and early detection
- Informing women about disease treatment and progression
- Being an advocate and resource for community referrals

Patient Education—Normal Menstrual Cycle

Average Menstrual Cycle

- Every 28 days; 14 days after ovulation; duration 5 days
- Approximate blood loss 50 mL

GYN BASICS

- Controlled by the following feedback mechanisms:
  - Hypothalamic-pituitary cycle
  - Ovarian cycle
  - Endometrial cycle

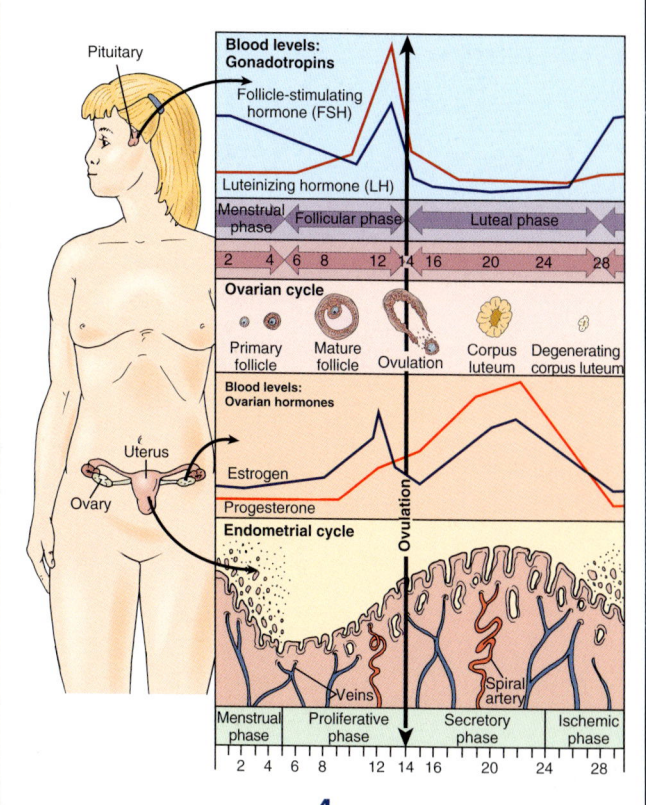

Pituitary

Uterus

Ovary

Blood levels: Gonadotropins

Follicle-stimulating hormone (FSH)

Luteinizing hormone (LH)

Menstrual phase | Follicular phase | Luteal phase

2 4 6 8 12 14 16 20 24 28

Ovarian cycle

Primary follicle | Mature follicle | Ovulation | Corpus luteum | Degenerating corpus luteum

Blood levels: Ovarian hormones

Estrogen

Progesterone

Ovulation

Endometrial cycle

Veins | Spiral artery

Menstrual phase | Proliferative phase | Secretory phase | Ischemic phase

2 4 6 8 12 14 16 20 24 28

Hypothalamic-Pituitary Cycle

- ↓ Estrogen and progesterone stimulate the hypothalamus to secrete gonadotropin-releasing hormone (GnRH)
- ↑ GnRH stimulates the anterior pituitary to secrete follicle-stimulating hormone (FSH)
- ↑ Levels of FSH stimulate development of the ovarian graafian follicles, which ↑ ovarian production of estrogen
- Midcycle, a slight ↓ estrogen triggers GnRH to stimulate the anterior pituitary to secrete luteinizing hormone (LH)
- A surge of LH and small ↑ in estrogen stimulate the graafian follicle to release an ovum (ovulation), changing the follicle into the corpus luteum. If fertilization does not occur, levels of estrogen and progesterone decrease and the corpus luteum regresses

Ovarian Cycle

- Follicular phase
  - Before ovulation 1–30 follicles begin to develop under the influence of FSH and estrogen
  - Under the influence of LH, one oocyte completes maturation and is released from the follicle
- Luteal phase
  - Begins after ovulation and ends with menstruation
  - Corpus luteum secretes estrogen/progesterone, peaks on day 8
  - Corpus luteum regresses without conception

Endometrial Cycle

- Menstrual phase (day 1–5)
  - Shedding of the functional $^2/_3$ of endometrium
- Proliferative phase (day 5–ovulation)
  - Rapid endometrial growth, influenced by estrogen
- Secretory phase (ovulation to 3 days before menses)
  - Endometrium thickens with ↑ blood and glandular secretions influenced by progesterone
- Ischemic phase
  - Spasm and necrosis of the functional layer of the endometrium

Gynecological Health

American Congress for Obstetricians and Gynecologists (ACOG) Guidelines for Cervical Cancer Screening

- Method: Liquid-based or conventional fixed-slide method of collecting exfoliated cervical cells from the cervical transformation zone with or without human papillomavirus (HPV) screen

Guidelines for average-risk women:

- Initial cervical screening should begin at age 21 years
- Women 21–29 years of age
  - Cervical cytology every 3 years
- Women 30–65 years of age
  - Cervical cytology with HPV test every 5 years (preferred), *or*
  - Cervical cytology alone every 3 years (adequate)
- Women 65 years or older. Stop screening if:
  - No history of cervical dysplasia
  - Three negative cytology results in a row
  - Two negative co-tests in a row in the past 10 years (most recent negative test performed in the last 5 years)
- Annual health promotion gynecologist visits

Sexual Health

Nurses can promote risk reduction measures intended to decrease the incidence of sexually transmitted infection (STI):

- Encourage the reduction of the number of sexual partners and mutually monogamous sexual relationships
- Encourage consistent and proper use of female and male condoms
- Encourage open discussion about sexual history and STI history with sexual partners
- Encourage screening and prompt treatment for STIs
- Discourage sexual activity until treatment is completed
- Encourage pre-exposure vaccination for vaccine-preventable STIs

CDC 2016 Adult Immunization Table

Vaccine▼ Age Group▶	19-21 years	22-26 years	27-49 years	50-59 years	60-64 years	≥65 years
Influenza*	1 dose annually					
Tetanus, diphtheria, pertussis (Td/Tdap)*	Substitute Tdap for Td once, then Td booster every 10 yrs					
Varicella*	2 doses					
Human papillomavirus (HPV) Female*	3 doses	3 doses				
Human papillomavirus (HPV) Male*	3 doses					
Zoster					1 dose	1 dose
Measles, mumps, rubella (MMR)*	1 or 2 doses depending on indication					
Pneumococcal 13-valent conjugate (PCV13)*						1 dose
Pneumococcal 23-valent polysaccharide (PPSV23)	1 or 2 doses depending on indication					1 dose
Hepatitis A*	2 or 3 doses depending on indication					
Hepatitis B*	3 doses					
Meningococcal 4-valent conjugate (MenACWY) or polysaccharide (MPSV4)*	1 or more doses depending on indication					
Meningococcal B (MenB)*	2 or 3 doses depending on vaccine					
Haemophilus influenzae type b (Hib)*	1 or 3 doses depending on indication					

Recommended for all persons who meet the age requirement, lack documentation of vaccination, or lack evidence of past infection; zoster vaccine is recommended regardless of past episode of zoster

Recommended for persons with a risk factor (medical, occupational, lifestyle, or other indication)

No recommendation

*Covered by the Vaccine Injury Compensation Program

Report at clinically significant postvaccination reactions to the Vaccine Adverse Event Reporting System (VAERS). Reporting forms and instructions on filing a VAERS report are available at www.vaers.hhs.gov or by telephone, 800-822-7967.

Information on how to file a Vaccine Injury Compensation Program claim is available at www.hrsa.gov/vaccinecompensation or by telephone, 800-338-2382. To file a claim for vaccine injury, contact the U.S. Court of Federal Claims, 717 Madison Place, N.W., Washington, D.C. 20005; telephone, 202-357-6400.

Additional information about the vaccines in this schedule, extent of available data, and contraindications for vaccinations is also available at www.cdc.gov/vaccines or from the CDC-INFO Contact Center at 800-CDC-INFO (800-232-4636) in English and Spanish, 8:00 a.m. - 8:00 p.m. Eastern Time, Monday-Friday, excluding holidays.

Use of trade names and commercial sources is for identification only and does not imply endorsement by the U.S. Department of Health and Human Services.

The recommendations in this schedule were approved by the Centers for Disease Control and Prevention's (CDC) Advisory Committee on Immunization Practices (ACIP), the American Academy of Family Physicians (AAFP), the American College of Physicians (ACP), the American College of Obstetricians and Gynecologists (ACOG) and the American College of Nurse-Midwives (ACNM).

Source: Department of Health and Human Services Centers for Disease Control and Prevention. Recommendations and Guidelines: Adult immunization schedule—United States, 2016. Retrieved from http://www.cdc.gov/es/schedules/downloads/adult/adult-pocket-size.pdf.

GYN BASICS

Common Sexually Transmitted Infections

For 2015 CDC Sexually Transmitted Disease Treatment Guidelines, visit http://www.cdc.gov/std/tg2015/default.htm.

Infection	Symptoms/Detection	Pregnancy Considerations
Chlamydia Most frequently occurring bacterial STI in the United States Screening recommended for women <25 years of age and older women at increased risk Incubation period 7–21 days	**Symptoms** • Often asymptomatic • Mucopurulent discharge • Postcoital bleeding • Dyspareunia • Abdominal pain • Dysuria **Detection** • Endocervical culture • Urine test	• Screen all pregnant women • Avoid doxycycline in pregnancy • Test of cure 3–4 weeks after treatment **Maternal Concerns** • Preterm labor • Premature rupture of membranes (PROM) • Postpartum endometritis **Neonatal Concerns** • Ophthalmia neonatorum (conjunctivitis) • Neonatal pneumonia
Gonorrhea Antimicrobial resistance demonstrated–refer to HYPERLINK "http://www.cdc.gov/std/tg2015/default.htm" CDC Treatment Guidelines Incubation period 2–10 days	**Symptoms** • Often asymptomatic • Purulent vaginal discharge • Dyspareunia • Abdominal pain • Dysuria **Detection** • Endocervical culture • Urine test	• Screen all pregnant women • Avoid quinolones or tetracycline **Maternal Concerns** • Preterm birth • PROM • Postpartum endometritis **Neonatal Concerns** • Ophthalmia neonatorum • Sepsis, subsequent arthritis, meningitis

Continued

Common Sexually Transmitted Infections—cont'd

Infection	Symptoms/Detection	Pregnancy Considerations
Hepatitis B Incubation period: 6 weeks to 6 months	**Symptoms** • Fatigue • Nausea/anorexia • Dark urine • Clay-colored stool • Jaundice/abdominal pain **Detection** • Serological testing • With acute infection:	• Screen all pregnant women **Neonatal Concerns** • CDC recommends administration of hepatitis B immunization to all newborns with birth weight >2000 g before hospital discharge • Infants born to HBsAg-positive mothers should have postexposure immunoprophylaxis

Test	Result
HBsAg	Positive
Total anti-HBc	Positive
IgM anti-HBc	Positive
Anti-HBs	Negative

Continued

Common Sexually Transmitted Infections—cont'd

Infection	Symptoms/Detection	Pregnancy Considerations
Herpes Simplex Virus (HSV) Incubation period: 2–10 days	**Symptoms** • Recurrent, painful vesicular lesions • Fever, malaise • Enlarged lymph nodes **Detection** • Cell culture and PCR	**Maternal Considerations** • Transmission to newborn greatest with primary infection • Cesarean birth recommended if active lesion in labor • Preterm labor **Neonatal Considerations** • Disseminated infections • CNS involvement • Localized infections of skin, eye, mouth
HIV Incubation period: 2 weeks to 6 months	**Symptoms** • Fever • Malaise • Lymphadenopathy • Skin rash • Rapid weight loss • Night sweats **Detection** • Antibody immunoassay • Rapid oral screen • Serum screen • Positive screen must be confirmed by more specific test, (Western blot or immunofluorescence assay)	• Routes of maternal-neonatal transmission • Transplacentally • Birth secretions • Breast milk • Transmission rate • Approximately 30% without treatment • 5%–8% w/antiretroviral therapy • 2% w/antiretroviral therapy + scheduled cesarean birth + avoidance of breastfeeding • Screen all pregnant women • Notify and counsel importance of testing in pregnancy

Continued

Common Sexually Transmitted Infections—cont'd

Infection	Symptoms/Detection	Pregnancy Considerations
Human Papillomavirus (HPV) HPV serotypes 16 and 18 have oncogenic potential and are linked to cervical cancer Incubation period: 3 weeks to 3 years	**Symptoms** • Often asymptomatic • Visible wart-like growths in genital area • Associated HPV serotypes 6 and 11 **Detection** • Physical examination • HPV-DNA test	**Maternal Concerns** • Decreased immunity may exacerbate viral infections • Genital warts may proliferate and become friable in pregnancy • Cesarean birth not routinely recommended solely for genital warts unless pelvic outlet is obstructed or increased risk for bleeding • Imiquimod, podophyllin, and podofilox not recommended in pregnancy **Neonatal Concerns** • May be linked with juvenile-onset respiratory papillomatosis
Syphilis Systemic disease caused by Treponema Pallidum Incubation period: 10-90 days	**Symptoms** • Primary syphilis: Chancre • Secondary syphilis: Skin rash, lymphadenopathy • Tertiary syphilis: Cardiac, ophthalmic, auditory involvement	**Maternal Considerations** • Uteroplacental transmission as high as 95% • Jarisch-Herxheimer reaction • May occur following treatment • Could precipitate premature labor and/or fetal distress

Continued

Common Sexually Transmitted Infections—cont'd

Infection	Symptoms/Detection	Pregnancy Considerations
Syphilis	**Detection** • Nontreponemal test (RPR/VDRL) • False-positive possible • $4\times \downarrow$ in titers indicate treatment success • Treponemal (FTA-ABS) • Specific for syphilis • Recorded as positive or negative	Symptoms • Acute febrile reaction • Headache • Myalgia **Neonatal Considerations** • Stillbirth • Congenital syphilis: Hepatosplenomegaly, jaundice, rhinitis, maculopapular rash, failure to thrive, chorioretinitis
Trichomoniasis Incubation period: 4–28 days	**Symptoms** • Frothy malodorous vaginal discharge • Dyspareunia • Vaginal itching/irritation • Dysuria **Detection** • Saline wet mount of vaginal discharge	**Maternal Concerns** • PROM • Preterm delivery **Neonatal Concerns** • Low birth weight

Breast Health Screening
  Method: Mammogram, Clinical Breast Exam, Breast Self-Awareness/Breast Self-Exam

ACOG guidelines for average-risk women:
- Annual mammogram starting at age 40 years
- Clinical breast exam by a health professional
  - Every 3 years from 20–39 years of age
  - Annual after age 40 years
- Discuss the benefits and limitations of breast self-awareness (BSA) and breast self-exam (BSE)

American Cancer Society guidelines for average-risk women (Revised 2015):
- Women aged 40–44 years should have the choice to start annual mammography
- Annual mammogram from age 45–54 years
- After age 55 years, a woman may choose to have mammography every 2 years

Instructions for Breast Self-Awareness (BSA) or Breast Self-Exam (BSE)
- BSA promotes a familiarity with how the breasts normally look and feel; women should notify their health-care provider if they notice:
  - Mass or thickening of the breast or axillary area
  - Edema, erythema, or warmth in the breast
  - Dimpling or scaly rash on the skin of the breast
  - Nipple discharge in a nonlactating woman
  - Sudden change in nipple or breast size or symmetry
  - Breast pain
- BSE is a systematic approach to examining the breast on a regular schedule

Instructions for Breast Self-Examination (BSE)

Step 1: Inspection
1. Visually inspect the breasts, looking for dimpling, lumps, skin irregularities, symmetry, or nipple discharge
2. Visually inspect in several positions; may accentuate an abnormality
   - Hands at the side
   - Hands above the head
   - Hands pressed onto hips
   - Leaning over

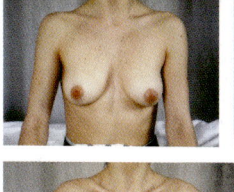
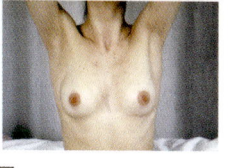
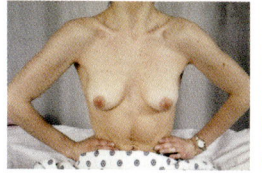
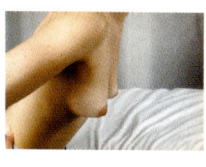

Step 2: Palpation

1. Feel the breast tissue and lymph node chain for lumps or thickening by using three finger pads while exerting light, medium, and deep pressure in a systematic fashion.
2. Begin by lying down on a flat surface with arm raised and a folded towel under the back on the side of the breast being examined.
3. After examining breast tissue, bring arm toward body and feel the axilla and the skin above as well as below the collarbone.
4. Repeat technique on the other breast.
5. Report lumps, thickening, nipple discharge, or any suspicious findings to health-care provider.

Preconception Counseling

Preconception counseling promotes healthy pregnancy and should be included for all women of childbearing age. The focus should be on factors that have an impact on organogenesis.

■ Discuss effects of ↑ maternal age on chromosomal abnormalities
■ Discuss the adverse effects of obesity on pregnancy outcome and make a plan for maintaining optimal weight
■ Encourage 400 mcg of folic acid daily to prevent neural tube defects

- Encourage intake of foods rich in folic acid
  - Enriched grain products
  - Fortified cereals
  - Leafy green vegetables
  - Beans
- Discourage use of alcohol, smoking, and drugs
- Teach about protection from sexually transmitted infections
- Update adult immunizations and investigate titers
- Review exposure to environmental risk factors
- Discuss control of chronic medical conditions
- Review safety of prescribed and over-the-counter (OTC) medications and herbs

Family Planning

Promote family planning:
- Educate women on available family planning methods, discussing the risks, benefits, and efficacy of each method
- Efficacy influenced by correct and consistent use, user preparedness, motivation, dexterity, and comorbidities

Sexual Abstinence

Refraining from sexual activity is the only 100% effective way to prevent pregnancy.

Fertility Awareness Methods

- Teach familiarity with body to recognize signs of fertility
- Are used to avoid or achieve pregnancy and to monitor gynecological health
- Advise couples to abstain during recognized period of fertility to avoid pregnancy

Evaluation of Cervical Mucus
- Amount and character of cervical mucus changes throughout the menstrual cycle in response to hormones
  - At ovulation, cervical mucus becomes more abundant, slippery, clear, and stretchable in response to estrogen (known as "spinnbarkeit")

- At ovulation, cervical mucus promotes sperm motility and ↑ probability of pregnancy with unprotected intercourse
- After ovulation, cervical mucus is scant, thick, cloudy, and no longer stretchable
- Women are taught to evaluate and chart cervical mucus daily

Basal Body Temperature (BBT)

- Monitor and graph BBT daily before rising
- Before ovulation, BBT decreases slightly in response to estrogen
- After ovulation, a surge of progesterone increases BBT by 0.5°–1.0°F
- BBT remains high with conception, but falls without conception, before menses
- Certain activities may alter BBT: smoking, use of electric blanket or heated waterbed, restless sleep, illness

Calendar Method

- Based on assumption that ovulation occurs 14 days before the onset of menses
- Record menstrual cycles for 6–8 months
- Calculate fertile period
  - Subtract 18 from the shortest menstrual cycle (28 − 18 = 10)
  - Subtract 11 from the longest menstrual cycle (32 − 11 = 21)
  - Days 10–21 fertile time; abstain from intercourse

Lactation Amenorrhea Method (LAM)

- Prolactin suppresses follicle-stimulating hormone (FSH), and therefore suppresses ovulation
- Postpartum women who exclusively breastfeed during the first 6 months after childbirth, including at least one night feeding, may postpone ovulation
- Instruct patients that ovulation and return of fertility may occur before first menses with a risk for unintended pregnancy

Barrier Methods

Barrier methods prevent conception by blocking entry of sperm into the cervix.

Diaphragm

- Dome-shaped rubber cup with a flexible ring that fits over the cervix; regularly examine integrity of rubber

- Inserted with spermicide applied to dome before intercourse and left in place for at least 6 hours after intercourse
- Should not be left in place more than 24 hours because of toxic shock syndrome risk
- Additional spermicide may be added with diaphragm still in place for repeated intercourse
- Diaphragm is custom fitted and must be refitted with 20-lb weight change and after a vaginal birth
- Urinary tract infections (UTIs) are more common with diaphragm use; teach to report symptoms of UTI
- Wash with soap and water after each use; inspect integrity of rubber by holding up to light to inspect for holes

Male Condom

- Thin latex sheath that covers the erect penis during sexual intercourse
- Condoms made of synthetic materials provide some protection from STIs
- Space should be left at the end of the condom for ejaculate
- Hold condom at base of the penis upon withdrawal to prevent spillage
- Only water-soluble gel should be used for lubrication to prevent degradation of the latex
- New condom should be used with each act of intercourse
- Store in unopened package in cool, dry place

Female Condom

- Prelubricated polyurethane sheath with two flexible rings
- Inner ring helps with insertion and covers the cervix
- Outer ring rests on vulva
- Water- or oil-based lubricant and spermicide may be used
- Can be stored at any temperature; 5-year shelf life
- Remove before standing by twisting the outer ring to contain semen and pull out
- Material degradation could occur if both male and female condoms are used simultaneously

Hormonal Methods

Hormonal contraceptives alter the normal menstrual cycle, inhibiting ovulation, altering the endometrial lining, and thickening cervical mucus.

Hormonal Contraceptives

- **Effects of Estrogen**
  - Ovulation inhibited by suppression of follicle-stimulating hormone (FSH) and luteinizing hormone (LH)
  - Endometrial lining altered, making the endometrium less receptive to implantation
- **Effects of Progestin**
  - Cervical mucus thickened, hampering sperm transport
  - Suppression of midcycle LH peak prevents ovulation
  - Decreased cilia movement within the fallopian tube

Advantages of Hormonal Contraceptives
- ↓ Dysmenorrhea
- ↓ Menstrual blood loss
- ↓ Endometrial/ovarian cancer

Disadvantages of Hormonal Contraceptives
- Requires addition of condom for STI protection
- Side effects may include the following:
  - Nausea/vomiting
  - Breast tenderness
  - Breakthrough bleeding
  - Headaches
  - Mood changes
  - Decreased libido
  - May cause serious health issues
- **REPORT** symptoms of possible complications, remember ACHES:
  - **A**bdominal pain
  - **C**hest pain
  - **H**eadache
  - **E**ye problems (blurred, double vision)
  - **S**evere leg pain, redness, and swelling
  - Shortness of breath
  - Worsening depression
  - Jaundice

Contraindications to Hormonal Contraceptives
- History of heart attack, stroke, blood clot; estrogen promotes blood clotting
- History of breast or female reproductive cancer; tumors may be hormonally provoked
- Diabetes with vascular involvement; estrogen promotes blood clotting

- Impaired liver function; metabolized through the liver and use may adversely affect existing liver disease
- Suspected or confirmed pregnancy
- Uncontrolled hypertension; increased risk for cardiovascular complications
- Smoker older than 35 years; increased risk for cardiovascular complications
- History of migraine headaches (with aura); increased risk for stroke
- Major surgery planned with immobilization; increased risk for deep vein thrombosis

Combination Hormonal Methods

Combination hormonal methods contain both an estrogen and progestin component.

Combination Oral Contraceptives (OCs)

- Most OCs are administered daily for 21 days, followed by 7 hormone-free days (either no pills taken or placebos taken for 7 days)
- Pill selection based on amount of estrogen, type of progestin, adrenergic effect, or symptoms presented
- Combined OCs may be monophasic (estrogen and progestin remain constant) or multiphasic (hormone dosing changes throughout the month)
- Extended-cycle OCs are taken consistently for 12 weeks, followed by 7 days of inert pills; withdrawal bleeding occurring only four times per year
- Combination hormonal contraceptives may decrease production of breast milk and should be avoided while breastfeeding
- Effectiveness of OCs are altered by certain medications; patients should report use of contraceptive agents to all health-care providers

Transdermal Patch

- Patch applied to skin weekly for 3 weeks; fourth week is patch free to allow withdrawal bleeding
- Acceptable application sites include abdomen, buttocks, upper outer arm, and upper torso (but not the breasts); site should vary weekly
- Application involves cleansing skin, avoiding lotion, and firmly applying patch, making sure all corners adhere to skin
- May engage in usual activities (bathing, swimming, exercising)
- Partial removal and skin reactions possible
- Decreased effectiveness noted in women who weigh more than 198 lb

GYN BASICS

- According to the U.S. Food and Drug Administration (FDA), women who use this method of birth control may be at an increased risk for venous thromboembolism; careful screening and counseling, weighing risk/benefits, should precede use

Vaginal Ring

- Small, flexible hormone-impregnated ring inserted and left in the vagina for 3 weeks; removed in fourth week to allow for withdrawal bleeding
- Ring should be kept inside unopened package before insertion; protect from sunlight and high temperatures
- Side effects include increase in vaginal discharge, vaginal irritation, or infection
- Expulsion may occur; if out for more than 3 hours, backup method of birth control needed for the next 7 days

Progestin-Only Preparations

- Progestin-only preparations are indicated for women who cannot use estrogen
- Alteration in menstrual cycle common with progestin-only methods
- May be used in lactation after breastfeeding is well established
- Side effects include weight gain, menstrual irregularities, and depression

Oral Contraceptives "Minipill"

- Compared with OCs that also contain estrogen, there is a greater risk for pregnancy if progestin-only pills are not taken at the same time each day
- Backup method of birth control needed with missed or late pills

Injectable Progestin Contraception: Depo-medroxyprogesterone (DMPA)

- Injected by health-care provider intramuscularly (IM) every 3 months
- Return to fertility may be delayed
- Bone loss may be of concern with continued use; alternative birth control method may be recommended after 2 years of continuous use

Implantable Progestins

- Matchstick-sized flexible implant inserted under the skin of the upper arm

- Protects against pregnancy for up to 3 years
- Inserted and removed by a health-care provider using local anesthesia
- Implant during the first 5 days of the menstrual cycle

Intrauterine System (IUS)/Intrauterine Device (IUD)

- Inhibits fertilization by altering fallopian tube transport of sperm and ova, in addition to producing cellular changes to the endometrial lining
- Inserted in office by qualified practitioner
- Increased incidence of pelvic inflammatory disease (PID)
- Uterine perforation and expulsion of device possible
- Attached to string that extends outside of the cervix; instruct patient to check for presence of string monthly
- Patient to REPORT signs of complications (remember PAINS):
  - **P**eriod late (pregnancy)
  - **A**bdominal pain (infection)
  - **I**nfection
  - **N**ot feeling well (infection)
  - **S**tring missing (IUD expelled)

Types
1. Hormone-releasing (levonorgesterol) device placed in the uterus to prevent pregnancy for 3–5 years, depending on type chosen
2. Copper IUD contains no hormones; continuous use for up to 10 years if no complications

Emergency Contraception

- Contraceptive agents used after unprotected intercourse intended for the prevention of pregnancy
- Available agents
  - Copper-T IUD
    - Inserted by health-care provider within 5 days of unprotected intercourse
  - Emergency oral contraceptive
    - Levonorgestrel oral contraceptives available OTC for women 17 years and older; state laws may vary
  - Ulipristal acetate (progesterone receptor modulator)
    - Best if used within 120 hours of unprotected intercourse

Permanent Birth Control Options for Women

- Prevent conception by mechanically blocking the fallopian tubes, preventing passage of ovum
- Low failure rate; however, if pregnancy occurs, may be ectopic

Tubal Ligation (Incisional Method)
- Performed in a hospital or outpatient surgical unit under general anesthesia
- Fallopian tubes cut, cauterized, and/or clipped
- Complications may include bleeding, infection, incomplete tube closure, injury to adjacent organs, or complications from anesthesia

Transcervical Tubal Sterilization (Nonincisional Method)
- Microinserts or tiny coils placed into the opening of the fallopian tubes, causing scar tissue to grow in approximately 3 months
- Performed in physician's office with local anesthetic
- Follow-up hysterosalpingogram performed at 3 months to ensure both tubes have been blocked; alternative method of birth control used until tube status verified
- Complications may include incorrect placement requiring second or operative procedure, ectopic pregnancy, infection, perforation of the uterus

Menopause

Menopause is the cessation of menses with amenorrhea for 12 months.

Symptoms

Vasomotor Symptoms
- Hot flashes
- Night sweats

Urogenital Symptoms
- Thin, friable vaginal mucosa
- Vaginal dryness and irritation
- Dyspareunia

Other Systemic Symptoms

- Sleep disturbance
- Mood swings
- Memory loss
- Skin changes
- Hair thinning

Hormone Replacement Therapy (HRT)

- The decision of whether to use hormone replacement therapy should be made after careful medical evaluation and discussion with the primary health-care provider concerning the risk/benefit ratio for each woman
- If HRT prescribed solely for vaginal/vulvar symptoms, local hormone therapy should be considered
- Alternatives to HRT should be considered if HRT used for sole purpose of osteoporosis prevention

Prevention and Treatment of Osteoporosis

- Risk factors for osteoporosis
  1. Menopause
  2. Low BMI
  3. Excessive caffeine use
  4. Smoking
  5. Sedentary lifestyle
  6. Family history
- Screening
  1. Fracture Risk Assessment Tool (FRAX)
  2. Dual-energy x-ray absorptiometry (DXA) scan of the spine and hip
     - Women age 65 years at average risk
     - High-risk women younger than age 65 years
  3. T-Score

Classification	T-Score
Normal	$\geq$−1.0
Osteopenia	−1.0 to −2.5
Osteoporosis	$\leq$2.5

■ Treatment
1. Lifestyle modification
   • Weight-bearing exercise
   • Postmenopausal intake of 1200 mg calcium daily
   • Vitamin D supplement
   • Smoking cessation
2. Biophosponates commonly prescribed to prevent bone loss
   • Take on an empty stomach
   • Sit up after taking medicine prescribed amount of time

Common Female Reproductive Disorders

Disorder	Presentation	Medical Treatment	Nursing Considerations
Cancer, Breast	• Breast mass • Nipple discharge • Dimpling • Nonpalpable mass detected by mammography	**Dx:** Biopsy, sentinel node biopsy **Treatment** • Lumpectomy • Mastectomy w/ reconstruction • Adjuvant therapy • Chemotherapy • Radiation • Aromatase inhibitors • Herceptin • Selective estrogen receptor modulators • Tamoxifen • Raloxifene	**Prognosis dependent on:** T: Tumor (size) N: Node (number involved) M: Metastasis **Lymphedema** • May occur after lymph node excision • Symptoms • Arm swelling • Feeling of tightness • Pain • Prevention (affected side) • No BP/IV venipuncture • Elevate limb • Encourage use of hand for eating, brushing hair
Cancer, Cervical	May be asymptomatic in early disease • Postcoital bleeding • Friable cervix • Abnormal Pap smear; may have evidence of HPV	**Dx:** Colposcopy with biopsy **Treatment** • LEEP • Cryosurgery • Hysterectomy • Chemotherapy • Internal radiation	• Early detection possible with cervical screening • Discuss HPV immunization for prevention

Continued

Common Female Reproductive Disorders—cont'd

Disorder	Presentation	Medical Treatment	Nursing Considerations
Cancer, Endometrial	May be asymptomatic in early disease • Abnormal uterine bleeding • Postmenopausal bleeding • Pelvic, back pain • Dyspareunia	**Dx:** Endometrial biopsy **Treatment** • Hysterectomy • Chemotherapy • Radiation	Posthysterectomy, REPORT: • Excessive bleeding • Difficulty urinating • Bowel dysfunction • Redness/drainage to incision • ↑Temperature
Cancer, Ovarian	May be asymptomatic in early disease **Triad of Symptoms** • Bloating • Increased abdominal size • Urinary frequency	**Dx:** Pelvic examination, ultrasound, laparoscopy with biopsy **Treatment** • Surgical excision • Radical hysterectomy • Chemotherapy • Radiation	Post-hysterectomy discharge teaching: • S/S menopause • Change in vaginal lubrication • Avoid heavy lifting, tub baths, tampons • Symptoms to report

Continued

Common Female Reproductive Disorders—cont'd

Disorder	Presentation	Medical Treatment	Nursing Considerations

Endometriosis	• Pain
	• Dysmenorrhea
	• Dyspareunia
	• Infertility
		Dx: Laparoscopy
		Treatment
		• Surgical excision
		• Medications
		• Androgen derivatives
		  • Side effects:
		    masculinizing traits,
		    weight gain, edema,
		    decreased breast
		    size
		• GnRH agonist
		  • Side effects: hot
		    flashes, vaginal
		    dryness, and bone
		    loss
		• Oral contraceptives
		• NSAIDs
			Action of GnRH/androgen
			derivate agonists:
			• Suppress ovulation
			• Shrink endometrial tissue
			• Prohibit further lesion
			  development

Continued

Common Female Reproductive Disorders—cont'd

Disorder	Presentation	Medical Treatment	Nursing Considerations

Pelvic Floor Dysfunction
• Uterine prolapse
• Rectocele
• Cystocele
	• Stress incontinence
	• Urgency
	• Constipation
	• Dyspareunia
	• Bulge at introitus
	• Dragging sensation
		Dx: Clinical presentation
		Treatment
		• Dependent on symptoms/grade of prolapse
		• Surgical
		  • Colporrhaphy
		  • Hysterectomy
		• Behavior modification
		  • Bladder/bowel training
		  • Knee-chest positioning
		  • Pelvic floor muscle training
			• Encourage Kegel exercises
			• Pessary
			• Ensure that patient can insert/remove
			• Teach to clean with soap/water
			• Perineum should be inspected for necrosis

Continued

Common Female Reproductive Disorders—cont'd

Disorder	Presentation	Medical Treatment	Nursing Considerations
Polycystic Ovarian Syndrome (PCOS)	• Irregular menses • Hirsutism • Obesity • Hyperinsulinemia • Hyperlipidemia • Hypertension • Infertility • Acne	**Dx:** Laboratory tests • FBS, HBA1C, lipid panel • Hormone level: testosterone, androgen, estrogen, prolactin, LH • Pelvic ultrasound **Treatment** • Medications • Metformin • Oral contraceptives	• Lifestyle modifications • Weight reduction • Exercise routine • Lower cholesterol
Uterine Fibroids	• Menorrhagia • Dysmenorrhea • Pelvic/rectal pressure • Dyspareunia • Urinary urgency	**Dx:** Ultrasound, hysteroscopy **Treatment** • Medications • Surgical • Uterine artery embolization • Myomectomy • Hysterectomy	Postembolization care: • Pain relief • Postembolization syndrome • Cramping • Nausea/vomiting • Fever • Lethargy • √ Groin for bleeding • √ Pedal pulse

Common Obstetrical Terms and Abbreviations

Term/Abbreviation	Definition
Abortion (Ab)	Spontaneous or induced termination of pregnancy before 20 weeks' gestation
ACOG	American Congress of Obstetricians and Gynecologists
AFP	Protein secreted by the fetus and found in maternal blood; maternal serum sample drawn between 15 and 18 weeks' gestation to detect babies with increased risk for neural tube defects or Down syndrome
Antepartum	Time of pregnancy
AWHONN	Association of Women's Health, Obstetric, and Neonatal Nurses
Chadwick's sign	Bluish hue of the cervix; probable sign of pregnancy
Chloasma	Deepening facial pigment resembling a mask related to increased estrogen levels
Colostrum	Breast fluid produced early in pregnancy and immediately after birth
C/S	Cesarean section; operative abdominal birth
Dilation	Opening of the cervical os
Effacement	Thinning of the cervix represented by percentage
Embryo	Human development in utero from day 15 until the 8th week of gestation
Ferning	Microscopic picture of amniotic fluid; resembles fern plant
Fetus	Developing baby in utero from 9 weeks' gestation until delivery
FHR	Fetal heart rate
Gestation	Time from conception to birth
Gestational diabetes	Glucose intolerance that is first recognized in pregnancy

ANTE-PARTUM

Common Obstetrical Terms and Abbreviations—cont'd

Term/Abbreviation	Definition
Goodell's sign	Softening of the cervix; probable sign of pregnancy
Gravid	Pregnant
Gravida (G)	Term used when counting the number of pregnancies
hCG	**H**uman **c**horionic **g**onadotropin
Hegar's sign	Softening of the lower uterine segment; probable sign of pregnancy
Lightening	Descent of the fetus into the birth canal
Linea nigra	Line of darkened pigmentation from the symphysis pubis to the umbilicus in pregnancy
LNMP	**L**ast **n**ormal **m**enstrual **p**eriod
Macrosomia	Large infant, greater than 4000 g (8.8 lb)
Missed abortion	Fetal demise without symptoms of cramping, bleeding, or dilation
Multiparity	Giving birth on multiple occasions
Neonate	First 28 days in the life of a newborn
NST	**N**onstress test
OTC	**O**ver-the-**c**ounter medications
Para (P)	Pregnancies that carry a fetus beyond 20 weeks' gestation
Placenta previa	Placenta that is implanted in the lower uterine segment, sometimes covering the cervical os
Postnatal	After birth
Prenatal	Before birth
Preterm labor	Initiation of labor between 20 0/7 and 36 6/7 weeks' gestation
Quickening	Fetal movement perceived by the mother, expected by 16 weeks' gestation

Continued

ANTE-
PARTUM

Common Obstetrical Terms and Abbreviations—cont'd

Term/Abbreviation	Definition
Round ligament pain	Occasional, sharp lower abdominal pain related to stretching of round ligament with uterine growth
Station	Relation of fetal presenting part with the maternal ischial spines
Striae	Stretch marks
Supine hypotension	Low blood pressure resulting from supine positioning in pregnancy; signs include pallor, nausea, diaphoresis, dizziness
Surfactant	A lipoprotein that maintains the stability of pulmonary tissue by reducing the surface tension
Teratogens	Substances that are harmful to the developing fetus; advise patient to avoid exposure
Term (T)	• Early term: 37 0/7 to 38 6/7 weeks' gestation • Full term: 39 0/7 to 40 6/7 weeks' gestation • Late term: 41 0/7 to 41 6/7 weeks' gestation • Postterm: ≥42 0/7 weeks' gestation
Threatened abortion	Symptoms of cramping and slight bleeding without cervical dilation in early pregnancy
Tocolytic	Medication given in an attempt to stop preterm labor

Confirming Pregnancy

- Pregnancy may be assumed based on the presence of certain signs and symptoms. *Presumptive* signs are subjective and recorded under the history of present illness
- *Probable* signs of pregnancy are assessed by the examiner and recorded as physical assessment findings
- *Positive* signs of pregnancy are those that are attributed only in the presence of a fetus

Presumptive	Probable	Positive
• Amenorrhea • Breast tenderness • Quickening • Nausea/vomiting • Urinary frequency	• Positive hCG • Uterine enlargement • Hegar's sign • Goodell's sign • Chadwick's sign	• FHR auscultated • Fetal movement palpated by health-care provider • Ultrasound of fetus

Urine Pregnancy Test

■ Reacts with human chorionic gonadotropin (hCG)
■ Performed on first voided urine sample of the day
■ Positive results possible before the first day of a missed menstrual period

Serum Pregnancy Test

■ Useful in monitoring expected pattern of progression of hCG
  ■ Qualitatively measures whether hCG is present
  ■ Quantitatively measures how much hCG is present
    • Should double every 48 hours in early pregnancy
    • Detects hCG as early as 9 days post-conception

Ultrasound

■ Confirms presence of gestational sac, fetal pole, and fetal cardiac activity in early pregnancy
■ Validates location of pregnancy (intrauterine versus ectopic)
■ Ultrasound measurement during the first trimester is the most accurate method to establish estimated due date

Estimated Date of Delivery

■ Establishing an accurate date of delivery is important to:
  ■ Determine timing of antenatal screening
  ■ Monitor growth of the fetus
  ■ Scrutinize timing of delivery

- Common abbreviations denoting delivery date
  - EDD: Estimated date of delivery
  - EDC: Estimated date of confinement
  - EDB: Estimated date of birth

Naegele's Rule

- Formula used to estimate date of delivery
- Count back 3 months and add 7 days to the last normal menstrual period (LNMP) reported by the patient
  - *Example:* The patient states that her LNMP was April 20th

$$\frac{4\text{th month (April)}\quad 20\text{th day}}{-3\,\text{months}\qquad +7\,\text{days}}$$
$$\text{1st month}\qquad 27\text{th day}$$

The baby is estimated to be due on January 27th of the following year.

Trimesters of Pregnancy

Normally, pregnancy continues for 40 weeks or 280 days
- 1st trimester: Conception until 13 weeks' gestation
- 2nd trimester: 14 weeks until 26 weeks' gestation
- 3rd trimester: 27 weeks until 40 weeks' gestation

Schedule of Prenatal Visits (low-risk pregnancy)

- Monthly until 28 weeks' gestation
- Biweekly from 28 weeks until 36 weeks
- Weekly from 36 weeks until delivery

Gathering a Prenatal Health History

Performing a thorough health history in the prenatal period is essential to planning nursing care and identifying high-risk women.
- Medical history
  - Chronic illness
  - Current and recent medication
  - Recent acute illness
  - Childhood illnesses

- Surgical history
  - Problems with anesthesia
  - Previous surgeries
  - Uterine/cervical surgeries
- Obstetrical history
  - Type of deliveries: vaginal/cesarean
  - Complications with past pregnancies
  - Infertility
  - Five-digit documentation of obstetrical history:

Descriptive Term	Definition
Gravidity (G)	Number of pregnancies
Term (T)	Deliveries ≥37 completed weeks
Preterm (P)	Deliveries >20 weeks but <38 weeks
Abortion (Ab)	Deliveries <20 weeks, spontaneous or induced
Living (L)	Number of living children

- *Documentation Example 1:* The prenatal client reports having three children at home. She states that her son was born on his due date, but her daughters were both born a month early. She reports that she lost a baby in her second month.
  - G: 5 (currently pregnant, 3 children at home, one abortion)
  - T: 1 (her son was born on his due date)
  - P: 2 (her daughters were each born a month early)
  - A: 1 (she lost a pregnancy at approximately 8 weeks)
  - L: 3 (reports three children at home)

Document as G5-1213

- Two-digit documentation of obstetrical history:
- *Documentation Example 2:* The same prenatal client may also be described as G5 (5 pregnancies) P3 (number of pregnancies that have reached 20 weeks); pregnancies ended before 20 weeks are not counted as "P" in this method.

Document as G5P3

- Sexual history
  - Number of sexual partners
  - Sexually transmitted infections
  - Sexual abuse
  - Methods of contraception
  - Condom use
- Social history
  - Use of recreational drugs
  - Smoking

- Domestic abuse
- Educational level/ability to read
- Economic status
- Type of health insurance
- Need for community referrals
- Transportation
- Nutrition
- Medications

Hormonal Changes in Pregnancy

Hormone		Functions
Estrogen	↑	Increases uterine muscle mass Increases blood flow to uterus Prepares breasts for lactation
Progesterone	↑	Relaxes venous walls Inhibits uterine contractions
hCG	↑	Stimulates estrogen/progesterone production
Relaxin	↑	Discourages uterine contraction Remodeling of collagen
Prolactin	↑	Maturation of breast ducts/alveoli Stimulates lactation
Human placental lactogen	↑	Insulin antagonist Allows adequate glucose for fetal demand

Nursing Care During the First Prenatal Visit

- Determine EDD based on LNMP
- Document current gestational age
- Document baseline vital signs
- Document height and weight and calculate body mass index (BMI)
- Obtain urine specimen and test for presence of:

Substance	Expected Finding
Glucose	Negative/trace
Protein	Negative/trace

- Auscultate fetal heart tones
- Measure fundal height in centimeters
  - Measure from the symphysis pubis to the top of the fundus
  - Uterine size increases in pregnancy in a predictable pattern and is measured to gauge fetal growth
  - Fundal height that is lagging or greater than expected should be further investigated

Gestational Age	Fundal Height
12	Just above symphysis pubis
16	Halfway between symphysis pubis and the umbilicus
20	At the umbilicus
21–36	Fundal height generally matches weeks of gestation in centimeters until 36 weeks; after lightening occurs and the fetus drops into the pelvis, there is a ↓ in fundal height

- *Example:* Fundal height at 28 weeks should be approximately 28 cm from the symphysis pubis

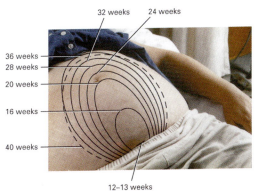

Fundal height.

Laboratory Tests

Common Laboratory Tests	Expected Finding in Pregnancy
HIV*	Negative
Blood type	A, B, AB, O
Rh factor	Negative or positive
Antibody screen	Negative
Hemoglobin	>11.5 mg/dL
Hematocrit	>33%
Platelets	150,000–400,000 mm³
WBC	5,000–12,000 mm³
RPR	Negative
Hepatitis B antigen	Negative
Rubella titer	1:8 immune
Hemoglobin electrophoresis	AA, unaffected
Chlamydia culture	Negative
Gonorrhea culture	Negative
Pap smear	Normal cytology

*ACOG recommends that all pregnant women be screened for HIV infection, as part of routine prenatal laboratory tests early in the pregnancy and repeated in the third trimester for women at high risk. Explanation of HIV infection, perinatal disease transmission, and benefits of treatment in pregnancy should be discussed.

Physiological Changes

↓ Heart rate	↓ Glomerular filtration rate
↑ Cardiac output	↑ Urine output
↑ Blood volume	↑ Basal metabolic rate
• Blood pressure (slight ↓ with return to baseline by 3rd trimester)	• Respiratory rate (no change)
↓ Systemic vascular resistance	↑ Stroke volume

↑ = Increase ↓ = Decrease

Diagnostic Testing in Early Pregnancy

Diagnostic Test	Nursing Considerations

Ultrasound
Clinical Applications:
• Confirm and date pregnancy
• Verify intrauterine pregnancy
• Detect fetal cardiac activity
• Measure fetal growth
• Detect fetal anomalies
• Measure amniotic fluid volume
• Determine fetal position
• Determine placental position
• Assess placental functioning
• Measure cervical length
• Measure nuchal translucency
• Adjunct to invasive procedures
	• Position to avoid supine hypotension; place rolled towel under right hip to move gravid uterus off inferior vena cava
	• S/S of supine hypotension
	  • Pallor
	  • Nausea
	  • Diaphoresis
	  • Tachycardia

Chorionic Villi Sampling (CVS)
Clinical Applications:
• Chromosomal analysis
• 10–12 weeks' gestation
	• ✓ Blood type, Rh, and antibody status
	• Administer Rh (D) immune globulin if indicated
	• Assess post-procedure
	  • ✓ Cramping
	  • ✓ Bleeding
	  • Monitor FHR

Continued

Diagnostic Testing in Early Pregnancy—cont'd

Diagnostic Test	Nursing Considerations

Amniocentesis
Clinical Applications:
• Chromosomal analysis
• Directly measure AFP
• Measure bilirubin level for fetal hemolytic disease
• Determine lung maturity by measuring surfactant
• Lecithin/sphingomyelin (L/S)
• Phosphatidylglycerol (PG)
	• √ Blood type, Rh, and antibody status
	• Administer Rh (D) immune globulin if indicated
	• Assess post-procedure
	  • √ Cramping
	  • √ Bleeding
	• Monitor FHR
	• Surfactant production must be sufficient before fetal lungs are considered mature
	• L/S ratio of 2:1 and + PG indicative of fetal lung maturity

Fetal Nuchal Translucency • Ultrasound measurement of back of fetal neck • Performed at 10–14 weeks Clinical Application: • Used in conjunction with maternal serum biomarkers to calculate risk for fetal chromosomal abnormality	Recommendations: • Used in conjunction with serum biomarkers for Down syndrome to calculate risk

Continued

Diagnostic Testing in Early Pregnancy—cont'd

Diagnostic Test	Nursing Considerations
Sequential Integrated Screening (SIS) • Pregnancy-associated placental protein A (PAPP-A) • Performed at 10–13 weeks • Nuchal translucency • Performed at 10–14 weeks	• Combines the results of markers in both the first and second semesters to determine risk for neural tube defects/Down syndrome/trisomy 18 • SIS using multiple markers increases the detection rate for Down syndrome by >90%, decreasing the number of pregnant women referred for invasive diagnostic testing
Maternal Serum Triple/Quad Screen • Measures AFP, hCG, estriol, inhibin levels • Performed at 15–18 weeks **Clinical Application:** • Maternal serum screen for neural tube defects/Down syndrome	• Results are adjusted according to: • Gestational age • Maternal age • Race • Weight • Presence of diabetes • Multiple gestation • Interpreting results: This is a screening method only. A positive result suggests the need for diagnostic testing with either amniocentesis or CVS and referral for genetic counseling

Education in the Early Prenatal Period

- Elevated estrogen and progesterone levels in early pregnancy generate changes in the body, causing pregnancy-associated discomforts; offer suggestions to lessen discomforts.
- Provide appropriate education for gestational age
- Teach patient to report symptoms that may indicate a potential complication (in red)

Discomfort	Patient Education
Breast discomfort	Hormone-related breast development often first presumptive sign of pregnancy • Encourage a supportive bra • Colostrum may be expressed in pregnancy • Introduce the value of breastfeeding • Introduce/reinforce breast self-examination Report any breast lump or unusual discharge
Emotional lability	Related to hormone changes • Discuss normalcy of emotional changes with patient and partner • Ambivalence normal in first trimester Report constant crying, inability to care for self, suicidal thoughts
Fatigue	Related to rapid hemodynamic and metabolic changes in the first trimester • Encourage naps during the day • Encourage prenatal vitamins • Encourage healthy diet Report syncope and vertigo
Leukorrhea	Related to vasocongestion of mucous membranes • Avoid tampon use and douching • Wear peri-pad to absorb discharge • Encourage cotton underwear Report vaginal discharge with an odor or color, vaginal bleeding, or leaking of amniotic fluid

Continued

42

Discomfort	Patient Education
Nasal stuffiness Epistaxis	Related to vasocongestion of mucous membranes • Increased humidity in home may help • Warm compresses to sinus area • Avoid OTC cold remedies unless prescribed Report fever, green/yellow nasal discharge, or frequent nosebleeds
Nausea and vomiting	Related to elevated hormone levels • Encourage small, frequent meals • Eat crackers before rising • Avoid pungent odors, spicy or greasy food • Discuss limited time frame for nausea • Subsides at approximately 12 weeks' gestation Report excessive vomiting
Urinary frequency	Related to uterine position/weight • Encourage frequent emptying of bladder • Discourage limiting oral fluids Report burning or pain with urination

■ Teach patient to avoid teratogens

Teratogen	Patient Education
Viruses	• Avoid contact with ill persons Infections causing serious harm to fetus: • **T**oxoplasmosis • **O**ther (hepatitis B) • **R**ubella • **C**ytomegalovirus • **H**erpes simplex virus (HSV) Report fever, rash, illness to primary health-care provider
Environmental	Avoid exposure to: • Mercury • Radiation • Lead • Other known environmental toxins

Continued

ANTE-PARTUM

Teratogen	Patient Education
Drugs and medications	
• Illicit drugs	• Assess use of alcohol, smoking, and illicit drugs • Discuss adverse effects to fetus • Encourage cessation of alcohol, smoking, and drugs • Refer to smoking cessation classes • Refer to addiction counselors, AA • Follow up on positive drug screens
• OTC/herbal	• Caution patient to discuss use of all OTC/herbals with primary health-care provider
• Prescription	• List name/dosage of all medications taken since LMP • Investigate drug safety • Medications in pregnancy should be prescribed after carefully weighing risks/benefits to the mother and fetus • FDA 2015 new drug labeling rule requires manufacturers to include risk summary, clinical considerations, and data in the following categories: • Pregnancy risk • Lactation • Females and males of reproductive potential

Health Maintenance

- Immunizations Recommended in Pregnancy (CDC Guidelines) Web link listed below
- Inactivated influenza vaccine (injectable)
- Tdap between 27 and 36 weeks' gestation
- Source: http://www.cdc.gov/vaccines/adults/rec-vac/pregnant.html

Nutrition

- Inquire about dietary practices
- Gather 24-hour diet recall

- Suggest an addition of 300 healthy calories per day
- Encourage daily prenatal vitamin with 400 mcg folic acid
- Foods rich in folic acid include:
  - Enriched grain products
  - Fortified cereals
  - Leafy green vegetables
  - Beans
- Teach food safety
  - Wash hands before and after food preparation
  - Thoroughly cook all eggs, meat, and seafood
    - Avoid unpasteurized dairy products and soft cheese
    - Avoid hot dogs and lunch meats unless heated until steaming hot
    - Avoid large fish (shark, swordfish, mackerel) known to contain high levels of mercury
- Suggest 6–8 glasses of water daily

Weight Gain in Pregnancy

- Recommended weight gain depends on prepregnancy weight/BMI

Prepregnant Weight	BMI	Recommended Total Weight Gain
Underweight	<18.5	28–40 pounds
Normal	18.5–24.9	25–35 pounds
Overweight	25–29.9	15–25 pounds
Obese	>30.0	11–20 pounds

- Assess and document the pattern of weight gain

Trimester	Suggested Weight Gain
1st	1–4 pounds total
2nd and 3rd	0.5–1 pound per week

Exercise in Pregnancy

- Physical activity in pregnancy is recommended unless contraindicated by medical complications

- Avoid sports with potential for abdominal trauma or falls
- Avoid overheating and supine positioning
- STOP exercise if experiencing:

■ Vaginal bleeding ■ Cramping ■ Leaking of amniotic fluid ■ Decreased fetal movement ■ Dizziness	■ Headache ■ Chest pain ■ Calf pain ■ Dyspnea

Sexuality in Pregnancy

- Sexual activity is not restricted in pregnancy unless risk factors exist for bleeding or preterm labor
- Discuss expected changes in sexuality
- Change in libido
- Body image changes
- Braxton-Hicks contractions with orgasm
- Comfortable positioning for intercourse

WARNING SIGNS DURING PREGNANCY

Patient should be instructed to notify primary health-care provider if experiencing any of the following symptoms:

Warning Sign	Possible Cause
Vaginal bleeding	Abortion Placenta previa Abruptio placentae Preterm labor
Leakage of vaginal fluid	Premature rupture of amniotic fluid Incontinence of urine
Dysuria	Urinary tract infection
Headache	Pregnancy-induced hypertension (PIH)

Continued

Warning Sign	Possible Cause
Altered vision Blurred vision Flashes of light	Pregnancy-induced hypertension (PIH)
Abdominal cramping	Preterm labor
Severe epigastric pain	Pregnancy-induced hypertension (PIH)
Decreased fetal movement	Fetal demise
Elevated temperature	Infection
Persistent vomiting	Hyperemesis gravidarum

Nursing Care for Return Prenatal Visits

- Measure pulse and blood pressure (BP)
- Compare BP to initial reading
- Measure in same position at each visit
- Measure weight and compare to last reading
- Note total weight gain
- Note pattern of weight gain
- Obtain urine specimen and test for protein and glucose
- Measure fundal height
- Determine fetal position
- Perform Leopold's maneuver
  - Palpate fetal body part in fundus (A)
  - Palpate for fetal back (B)
  - Palpate for presenting part (C)
  - Palpate for attitude of presenting part (D)

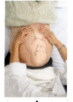 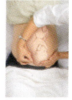 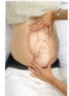

| A | B | C | D |

Leopold's maneuver.

- Place Doppler on maternal abdomen over fetal back to monitor fetal heart rate
- Record presence of fetal movement
- Assess for presence of edema/deep tendon reflexes
- Record symptoms since last visit
- Discuss procedure for diagnostic testing

Diagnostic Tests	Nursing Considerations
1-Hour Glucose Screen • Performed on all pregnant women at 24–28 weeks • Performed at first prenatal visit and repeated as needed at 24–28 weeks in women identified as high risk: • BMI ≥30 • Hx of gestational diabetes in previous pregnancy • Clinical Application: Detection of gestational diabetes	• Administer 50 g glucose load • Patient should not eat, drink, or smoke during the test • Serum sample drawn in 1 hour **Expected Result: ≤135–140 mg/dL**
Group B Vaginal Culture • Performed between 35 and 37 weeks • Clinical Application: Detects group B streptococcus in asymptomatic women	• Explain test to patient • Collect vaginal/rectal specimen • Positive culture treated with intravenous antibiotics in labor to prevent transmission to the newborn **Expected Result: Negative**
Fetal Fibronectin (fFN) • Performed between 22 and 35 weeks in women at high risk for preterm labor • Clinical Application: Negative predictive value for preterm labor	• NO intercourse for 24 hours before examination • Cervical/posterior fornix fluid collection • Result often combined with ultrasound measurement of cervical length **Expected Result: Negative**

Continued

Diagnostic Tests	Nursing Considerations
Antibody Screen • Performed at 28 weeks in Rh-negative women • Clinical Application: Detects presence of positive antibodies in serum of Rh-negative women	• Administer Rho (D) Immune Globulin at 28 weeks to prevent antibody formation if Rh negative and antibody screen negative **Expected Result: Negative**

Education in the Second and Third Trimesters

Fetal Kick Counts

- Count fetal movement daily
  - Find a comfortable position in a quiet place
  - Note the time started and count the number of fetal movements
  - Document time required for 10 movements
  - REPORT immediately if 10 movements are not achieved in 2 hours or if the pattern of fetal movement changes
- Discuss fetal growth and development
- Demonstrate palpation of the uterus for contractions
- Discuss symptoms of preterm labor
  - Lower backache
  - Increased vaginal discharge
  - Bloody show
  - Leaking amniotic fluid
  - Contractions
  - Pelvic pressure
- Differentiate between true and false labor:

True Labor	False Labor
Cervix dilates	Cervix unchanged
Contractions ↑ intensity/ frequency	Contractions ↓ with position/activity change Irregular
Loss of amniotic fluid Bloody show	No change in vaginal discharge

- Encourage childbirth preparation class
- Discuss options for pain control in labor
- Cesarean preparation class, if indicated
- Epidural anesthesia class, if indicated
- Explore preparing for the newborn
  □ Breastfeeding
  □ Circumcision
  □ Choosing a pediatrician
  □ Car seat safety
- Discuss the discomforts and expected body changes associated with late pregnancy and teach reportable symptoms (in red)

Discomfort	Patient Education
Backache	Related to shift in posture due to gravid uterus • Encourage low-heeled shoes • Avoid standing for long periods • Teach pelvic tilt exercises Report constant or rhythmic backache
Braxton-Hicks contractions	Instruct patient how to palpate for contractions • Labor symptoms should not be present until 39 weeks' gestation • Monitor for symptoms of labor Report signs of labor for prompt evaluation
Constipation, hemorrhoids	Related to decreased gastric motility; iron supplement may worsen constipation • Increase dietary fiber and water intake • Encourage exercise • Discourage enemas and laxatives Report painful or bleeding hemorrhoids
Faintness	Related to hemodynamic changes • Avoid sudden position change • Avoid long periods without eating • Avoid lying supine Report loss of consciousness

Continued

Discomfort	Patient Education
Heartburn	Related to increased pressure on abdominal organs and sphincter relaxation • Encourage small, frequent meals • Avoid spicy foods • Sit up after meals Report persistent symptoms
Insomnia	Related to fetal movement, nocturia • Teach relaxation techniques • Encourage side-lying with pillow support • Warm milk/shower before sleep
Leg cramps	Related to uterine pressure on the pelvic nerves or calcium imbalance • Review daily calcium intake • Teach signs of deep vein thrombosis Report pain, redness, localized heat
Peripheral edema	Related to venous return from pressure of the gravid uterus • Rest in lateral recumbent position • Elevate legs when sitting • Continue with 6–8 glasses water daily Report generalized edema
Pigmentation changes: • Linea nigra • Chloasma • Striae	Related to hormone changes in pregnancy • Fade after pregnancy • Moisturizers decrease itching, but will not prevent striae Report body rashes
Round ligament pain	Related to stretching of the round ligament with uterine growth and rotation • Change positions slowly • Encourage good body mechanics Report abdominal cramping, constant pain, or bleeding

Continued

ANTE-PARTUM

Discomfort	Patient Education
Shortness of breath	Related to upward diaphragmatic pressure exerted by the gravid uterus • Allow more time for strenuous activities • Eat small, frequent meals • Lightening will lessen symptoms Report unrelieved dyspnea with rest
Varicose veins	Caused by venous stasis related to pressure from the gravid uterus • Wear pregnancy support hose • Avoid lengthy standing • Change positions frequently Report pain, redness, localized heat to legs

Fetal Surveillance in Pregnancy

Nonstress Test (NST)

Procedure used to monitor fetal response to movement; FHR acceleration with fetal movement is reassuring and a sign of fetal well-being.
■ Place patient in a Semi-Fowler's or side-lying position
■ Record vital signs and apply electronic fetal monitor
■ Record baseline fetal heart rate and monitor pattern for minimum of 20 minutes (may take up to 40 minutes or longer to take into account the fetal sleep-wake cycle)
■ NST may take longer with absence of accelerations; fetal movement may be stimulated vibroacoustically
■ Report findings to primary health-care provider

Expected Findings—Reactive
Two accelerations of FHR within 20 minutes that are at least 15 BPM above the baseline rate and last for a minimum of 15 seconds each

Contraction Stress Test (CST)

Also called Oxytocin Challenge Test (OCT), the CST is a procedure used to determine fetal tolerance to the stress of uterine contractions.
■ Calculate gestational age (should not be performed on preterm patients; test stimulates contractions)

- Place patient in side-lying position
- Record vital signs
- Apply EFM and record baseline fetal heart rate for 20 minutes
- Stimulate uterine contractions until three contractions occur within 10 minutes lasting 40 seconds each
- Contractions can be stimulated with
  - Nipple stimulation *or*
  - IV Oxytocin per hospital protocol
- Document FHR response to contractions

Expected Finding—Negative

Three contractions that last at least 40 seconds within 10 minutes without the presence of late or significant variable decelerations

Biophysical Profile (BPP)

- Exam performed to assess fetal well-being
- Test includes ultrasound, observing four specific fetal criteria + NST included as a fifth parameter
- Scoring of Biophysical Profile (BPP):

Parameter Measured	Expected Findings (within 30 minutes)	Score
Fetal tone	1+ episodes of active limb or hand flexion/extension	2
Fetal breathing	1+ episodes lasting 30 seconds	2
Gross fetal movement	3+ discrete movements	2
Amniotic fluid volume	Pocket of amniotic fluid that measures at least 2 cm	2
NST	Reactive	2

Expected Finding—

Score of at least 8/10

Pregnancy Complications

Vaginal Bleeding (Before 20 Weeks' Gestation)

May be related to spontaneous abortion, ectopic pregnancy, or gestational trophoblastic disease.

Spontaneous Abortion

Loss of pregnancy before viability.

Clinical Findings

- Vaginal spotting (may pass clots)
- Abdominal cramping
- Cervical effacement/dilation
- Fetal heartbeat may be present or absent

Ectopic Pregnancy

Products of conception implant outside the uterus.

Clinical Findings

- Vaginal spotting
- hCG lower than expected for dates
- Lower abdominal pain

Ultrasound Findings

- Absence of intrauterine gestational sac

If Rupture Occurs

- Positive Cullen's sign (periumbilical bluish hue)
- Shoulder pain
- Signs of shock

Gestational Trophoblastic Disease

Abnormal proliferation of trophoblastic cells without viable fetus.

Clinical Findings

- Vaginal spotting (dark brown)
- Fundal height greater than expected for dates
- hCG greater than expected for dates
- Excessive nausea and vomiting
- Absence of fetal heart tones

Ultrasound Findings

- Snowflake-like clusters, absence of fetus

Nursing Care—Vaginal Bleeding in Early Pregnancy

- Monitor amount, color of bleeding
- Collect passed tissue/clots
- Assess vital signs
- Observe for signs of shock
- Assess for fetal heart rate
- Monitor patient comfort
- Provide pain medications as ordered

- Attend to patient's emotional needs
- View/report laboratory/ultrasound findings
- Check blood type and Rh factor
  - Administer Rh(D) immunoglobulin if indicated
- Monitor intake/output
- Initiate IV fluids as ordered
- Type and cross for blood products as ordered

Vaginal Bleeding After 20 Weeks' Gestation

Placenta Previa

Low-lying position of placenta in the uterus that partially or completely covers the cervical os.

Clinical Findings

- Painless bright red vaginal bleeding
- Bleeding may be reported after intercourse
- Uterine tone soft upon palpation

Nursing Interventions

Dependent on the following:

- Amount of bleeding
- Labor status
- Gestational age
- Fetal response
- If labor active and os is completely covered, C/S indicated
- If bleeding controlled and labor absent, conservative management
- **Conservative Management Teaching**
  - Activity limitation
  - No tampon use
  - No sexual intercourse
  - Monitor and report bleeding
  - Patient instructed to report placenta placement when admitted to hospital
  - Cesarean preparation class
- Count fetal movements

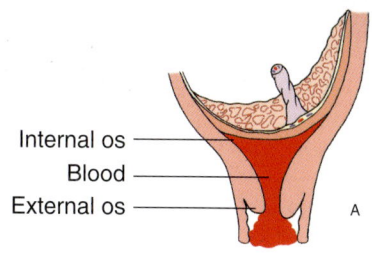

Internal os

Blood

External os

A

Complete placenta previa.

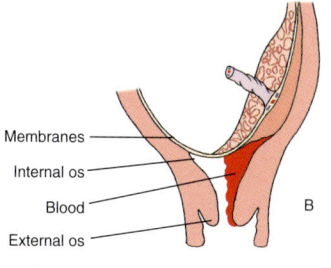

Membranes

Internal os

Blood

External os

B

Partial placenta previa.

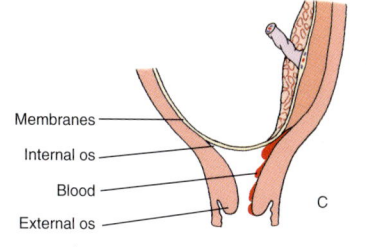

Membranes

Internal os

Blood

External os

C

Marginal placenta previa.

Abruptio Placentae

Premature separation of the placenta; may be partial or complete.

Clinical Findings

- Abdominal pain (sudden onset, intense and localized)
- Fundus firm, boardlike, with little relaxation
- Vaginal bleeding
- Bleeding may be concealed within the uterine cavity
- Alteration in FHR pattern

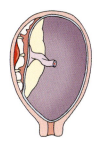
Partial separation
(concealed hemorrhage)

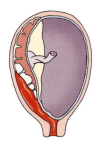
Partial separation
(apparent hemorrhage)

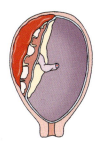
Complete separation
(concealed hemorrhage)

Nursing Care With Vaginal Bleeding in Late Pregnancy

- Monitor amount of bleeding
- Check vital signs
- Observe for signs of shock
- Evaluate fetal heart tones
- Palpate uterine tone
- Apply electronic fetal monitor (EFM)
- REPORT category II and III FHR patterns
- REPORT tachysystole
- Do not attempt vaginal examination until placenta placement verified
- Initiate IV fluids
- Report laboratory and ultrasound findings
- Prepare staff for possible cesarean birth
- Attend to patient's emotional needs

Hyperemesis Gravidarum

Intractable vomiting in pregnancy with resultant weight loss and dehydration; usually occurs in the first trimester.

Clinical Findings
- Inability to retain food and/or oral fluids
- Weight loss
- Fatigue

Nursing Care
- Assess vital signs
- Observe for signs of dehydration
- Review electrolytes
- Access IV site as ordered
- Record fetal heart rate pattern
- Record intake and output
- Record daily weight
- Check urine for ketones
- Administer antiemetics as ordered

Preterm Labor

Onset of labor before the 37th completed week of gestation.

Clinical Findings
- Rhythmic lower abdominal cramping
- Complaints of backache
- Increased vaginal discharge
- Downward pelvic pressure
- Leaking of amniotic fluid
- Vaginal spotting
- Cervical effacement/dilation
- Shortening cervical length

Nursing Care
- Determine gestational age
- Assess uterine tone and contraction status
- Auscultate fetal heart tones and apply EFM
- Assess for maternal infection
    - Obtain vaginal/urine cultures
    - Assess maternal temperature
    - Note color and odor of vaginal fluid

- Assess for presence of amniotic fluid
  - *Nitrazine paper:* Amniotic fluid has alkaline properties; nitrazine paper changes from yellow to blue
  - *Microscopic analysis:* Amniotic fluid resembles fern plant "ferning pattern"
  - *Speculum examination:* Assess for pooling of amniotic fluid
- Assess cervical dilation and effacement
- Position side-lying
- Initiate IV fluids as ordered
- Initiate corticosteroid as ordered
  - Accelerates fetal lung maturity
  - Greatest benefit 24-hours after administration
  - Given between 24–34 weeks' gestation
- Initiate tocolytic therapy as ordered

Tocolytic Medication	Nursing Precautions

Magnesium Sulfate
ANTIDOTE: Calcium gluconate at bedside
	• Monitor intake and output
	• Assess pattern of fetal heart rate
	• Monitor for contractions
	• Auscultate lungs
	• Report magnesium sulfate levels
	• Watch for signs of toxicity:
	  • Absence of deep tendon reflexes
	  • Respiration depression
	  • Decreased level of consciousness
	  • Decreased urine output

β-Adrenergic Agonist Terbutaline Ritodrine	• Monitor for hypotension • Assess for tachycardia • Assess patient for tremors • Assess for pulmonary edema • Screen glucose/potassium • Assess for cardiac arrhythmias/chest pain • Monitor pattern of fetal heart rate • Monitor contractions
Prostaglandin Antagonist Indomethacin	• May lead to premature constriction of ductus arteriosus
Calcium Channel Blockers Nifedipine	• Monitor for hypotension

Hypertensive Disorders in Pregnancy

Preeclampsia

Preeclampsia: Hypertension disorder of pregnancy recognized after 20 weeks' gestation with multisystem involvement

Clinical Findings
- Hypertension
  - BP of 140/90 mm Hg or higher
- Proteinuria and renal involvement
  - Dipstick urine of 1+ or more
  - 300 mg of protein in a 24-hour urine collection
  - Elevated serum creatinine
- Blurred or altered vision
- Epigastric pain
- Headache
- Edema
- Hyperreflexia

Eclampsia

Eclampsia: Severe preeclampsia complicated with new-onset convulsion
- Can occur during pregnancy or in the postpartum period
- Worsening of symptoms of preeclampsia
- Seizure activity

HELLP Syndrome

Clinical Findings
- Worsening symptoms of preeclampsia
- Malaise
- Epigastric pain
- Nausea/vomiting

Laboratory Findings
- **H**emolysis
- **E**levated **L**iver enzymes
- **L**ow **P**latelets

Nursing Care
- Closely monitor vital signs
  - Report worsening of symptoms
- Assess deep tendon reflexes
  - Report worsening hyperreflexia and clonus

- Monitor kidney function
  - Monitor intake and output
  - Collect 24-hour urine as ordered
  - Report abnormal renal function laboratory findings
- Assess for edema
  - Assess for upper body edema
  - Assess daily weight
  - Record intake and output
- Assess fetal status
  - Evaluate fetal heart rate (FHR) tracing
  - Report category II and category III FHR patterns
- Palpate tone of fundus
- Monitor patient comfort
- Place patient in side-lying position
- Keep environment quiet and dim
- Institute seizure precautions
  - Side rails up and padded
  - Bed in low position
  - Suction equipment available at bedside
  - Oxygen available at bedside
- Initiate IV fluids as ordered
- Initiate medications as ordered

Drug Therapy	Nursing Precautions
Magnesium sulfate	See precautions listed under preterm labor for magnesium sulfate
Antihypertensives	Administer slowly Closely monitor for hypotension

Gestational Hypertension

Gestational Hypertension: New-onset hypertension recognized after 20 weeks' gestation without symptoms of preeclampsia

Chronic Hypertension

Chronic Hypertension: Hypertension that predates pregnancy identified before 20 weeks' gestation

Gestational Diabetes

Clinical Findings

- Polyuria
- Polydipsia
- Polyphagia
- Fatigue
- Blurred vision
- Glucosuria
- Recurrent yeast infections
- Slow healing wounds

Abnormal glucose results:

1-hr glucose	≥135–140 mg/dL

Abnormal 3-hour glucose tolerance test if 2 of 4 of the following values are elevated:

FBS	<95 mg/dL
1-hr	<180 mg/dL
2-hr	<155 mg/dL
3-hr	<140 mg/dL

Nursing Care

- Dietitian consult for ADA diet instructions
- Discuss pathophysiology of gestational diabetes with patient
- Demonstrate home glucose monitoring
- Review range for glycemic control
- Demonstrate logging of glucose results
- Discuss role of exercise in glycemic control
- Demonstrate urine ketone testing
- Demonstrate insulin administration
- Teach patient to count fetal movement
- Teach patient about fetal surveillance testing
  - Nonstress test
  - Biophysical profile
  - Ultrasound
- Women with gestational diabetes should be screened at 6–12 weeks' postpartum for glucose impairment with a 75-g 2-hour OGTT

Common Intrapartum Terms and Abbreviations

Term/Abbreviation	Definition
Active labor	Second phase in the 1st stage of labor characterized by cervical dilation of 4–7 cm
AFI	Amniotic fluid index
Amnioinfusion	Installation of normal saline into the uterine cavity during labor to decrease the occurrence of cord compression and associated variable decelerations
AROM	**A**rtificial **r**upture **of m**embranes
Attitude	Relation of the fetal body parts to one another
Bishop's score	Set of criteria used to calculate cervical readiness for labor
BPP	**B**io**p**hysical **p**rofile; fetal well-being assessment
Breech presentation	Fetus positioned so that the buttocks or feet are the presenting part
Cardinal movements	Movements of the fetus when traveling through the birth canal
Cephalic presentation	Fetus positioned so that the fetal head is the presenting part; most common fetal position in utero
Dilation	Opening of the cervix caused by rhythmic uterine contractions; starts closed and opens to 10 cm
EDD	**E**stimated **d**ay of **d**elivery
Effacement	Shortening and thinning of the cervix
Effleurage	Rhythmic light stroking of the abdomen as a measure to decrease pain in labor
EFM	**E**lectronic **f**etal **m**onitoring
Engagement	Occurs when the fetal presenting part passes into the maternal true pelvis
FHR	**F**etal **h**eart **r**ate

Continued

Continued

Common Intrapartum Terms and Abbreviations—cont'd

Term/Abbreviation	Definition
Fetal attitude	Relation of the fetal body parts to each other; example: chin to chest (flexion)
Fetal lie	Relationship of the fetal spine to the maternal spine, most often longitudinal
Fetal presentation	The part of the fetus that is positioned closest to the cervix and is delivered first in a vaginal birth
Ferguson reflex	Maternal urge to push preceded by stretching of the posterior vagina and release of endogenous oxytocin
Friedman curve	Assessment tool that determines the normalcy of the progress of labor
Fundus	Uppermost portion of the uterus
Intrapartum	Time of labor and birth
IUPC	Intrauterine pressure catheter; internally measures uterine tone with contractions and rest
Kangaroo care	Skin-to-skin contact with mother and newborn
Latent labor	1st phase of the 1st stage of labor characterized by 0–3 cm cervical dilation
Leopold's maneuvers	Systematic palpation of the gravid abdomen to determine fetal position and expedite location of FHR
Lightening	Descent of the fetal presenting part into the pelvic cavity often 2 weeks before labor begins in primiparas
LOA	Left occiput anterior; referring to the relation of the fetal presenting part to the maternal pelvis
McRobeT's maneuver	Maternal positioning for pushing with shoulder dystocia; maternal legs flexed apart with knees placed onto abdomen

Common Intrapartum Terms and Abbreviations—cont'd

Term/Abbreviation	Definition
NST	Nonstress test
Para	Number of pregnancies that resulted in birth
Primipara	Woman who delivers one fetus to viability
PROM	Premature rupture of membranes
Station	Location of the presenting fetal part in relation to the maternal ischial spines
Tachysystole	>5 contractions in 10 minutes
Tocolytic agent	Medication used to decrease uterine contractions in preterm labor
Transition	Last phase of the 1st stage of labor characterized by contractions every 2–3 minutes lasting 90 seconds with cervical dilation of 8–10 cm
Turtle sign	Upon pushing, regression instead of forward movement of fetal head with subsequent contractions
VBAC	Vaginal birth after cesarean

Admission to Birthing Unit

Upon admission to labor and delivery, the nurse should:
- Determine reason for admission
- Gather patient history
- Review prenatal health record
- Perform a physical examination of mother and fetus

Prenatal History

- Estimated date of delivery (EDD)
- Current gestational age
- Complications in pregnancy

- Results of laboratory tests and ultrasounds
- Medications used in pregnancy
- Presence of vaginal discharge or bleeding
- Amniotic fluid status
- Presence of fetal movement
- Onset and pattern of contractions

Obstetrical History

- Length of labor
- Birth complications
- Neonatal outcomes
- Type of birth
  - Vaginal
    - Instrumentation
    - Episiotomy
  - Cesarean
    - Reason for cesarean
    - Type of incision
      - Low transverse
      - Classical

Medical History

- Chronic health problems
- Current medications
- Time and description of last oral intake
- Allergies to food/medicine

Surgical History

- Complications with anesthesia
- Date/reason/type of surgery

Performing a Physical Examination

- Assess maternal vital signs
- Collect urine specimen for protein and glucose
- Assess for presence of edema
- Assess deep tendon reflexes
- Perform Leopold's maneuver to determine fetal position (See *Antepartum* Tab, p. 47)
- Assess fetal heart rate (FHR)
- Measure fundal height (See *Antepartum* Tab, p. 37)
- Determine the frequency, duration, and intensity of contractions
- Determine the stage and phase of labor
  - Stage 1: Cervical dilation from 0–10 cm, divided into three phases
    - Latent phase: Cervix dilates 0–3 cm
    - Active phase: Cervix dilates 4–7 cm
    - Transition: Cervix dilates 8–10 cm
  - Stage 2: Complete cervical dilation until birth of the fetus
  - Stage 3: Birth of fetus until birth of placenta
  - Stage 4: First 2 hours of recovery after birth
- Assess cervical changes
  - Dilation (0–10 cm)
  - Effacement (0%–100%)
- Assess station

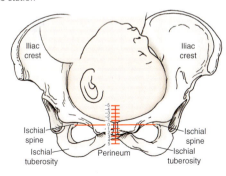

Station.

- Note presence, color, and amount of bloody show
- Check status of amniotic membranes
  - Intact
  - Bulging
  - Ruptured (note color, amount, and odor)
    - Confirming rupture of membranes (ROM)
      - *Nitrazine paper:* Amniotic fluid has alkaline properties; Nitrazine paper changes from yellow to blue
      - *Microscopic analysis:* Amniotic fluid resembles fern plant "ferning pattern"
      - *Speculum examination:* Assess for pooling of amniotic fluid

Nursing Responsibility With Fetal Monitoring

- Position to avoid supine hypotension
  - Rolled towel under right hip to move gravid uterus off of inferior vena cava
  - Side-lying
  - Semi-Fowler's
- Compare FHR to maternal pulse to ensure fetal assessment
- Review FHR pattern in conjunction with contraction pattern
- Determine whether FHR tracing is normal (category I), indeterminate (category II), or abnormal (category III)
- Implement nursing interventions and evaluate effectiveness for the identified category
- REPORT category II and category III FHR patterns to primary health-care provider
- Document findings and interventions using standardized descriptive terms
- Stay current with ongoing education and periodic competence validation

Three-Tier FHR Pattern Interpretation

Category	Definition	Indication
I Normal	All of the following must be present: • Baseline FHR 110–160 bpm • Moderate variability • No late or variable decelerations • May or may not exhibit early decelerations • May or may not exhibit accelerations	• Predictive of normal fetal acid-base balance • Routine follow-up to support labor

II
Indeterminate
	May include:
	• Baseline rate: Tachycardia or bradycardia (not accompanied by absent variability)
	• Variability: Minimal, marked, or absent (not accompanied by recurrent decelerations)
	• Accelerations: Not inducible with fetal stimulation
	• Periodic or episodic decelerations:
	  • Recurrent variable decelerations with minimal to moderate variability
	  • Prolonged decelerations
	  • Recurrent late decelerations with moderate variability
	  • Variable decelerations with slow return to baseline, overshoots or shoulders
		• Requires heightened surveillance
		• Support normal contraction patterns
		• Promote optimal fetal oxygenation
		• Ensure proper maternal positioning
		• Communicate changes to primary health-care provider

Continued

Three-Tier FHR Pattern Interpretation—cont'd

Category	Definition	Indication
III Abnormal	Absent variability plus: • Recurrent late decelerations • Recurrent variable decelerations • Bradycardia • Sinusoidal pattern	• Predictive of abnormal fetal acid-base balance • Requires prompt evaluation and action • Intrauterine resuscitation • Expeditious birth as appropriate

Types of Fetal Monitoring

Intermittent Auscultation

Auscultate fetal heart tone (FHT) over fetal back with Doppler or fetoscope.

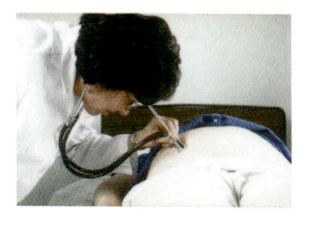

Fetoscope.

- Count FHR before and immediately after a contraction
- Note both FHR and rhythm
- Frequency of auscultation based on:
  - Phase/stage of labor
  - Hospital protocol
  - Risk status
  - Labor interventions
  - Physician orders

Stage/Phase of Labor	Frequency of FHR Monitoring
Stage 1: Latent phase	Every 30–60 minutes
Stage 1: Active phase	Every 15–30 minutes
Stage 1: Transition	Every 5–15 minutes
Stage 2: Pushing	Every 5–15 minutes

Continuous Fetal Monitoring
Monitored with external or internal fetal monitoring.

External Fetal Monitoring (EFM)
- Encourage patient to vcid before applying EFM
- Test internal circuitry of EFM
- Perform Leopold's maneuver
  - Place ultrasound transducer over fetal back
  - Place toco transducer over uterine fundus

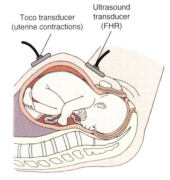

External fetal monitor.

Internal Fetal Monitoring
- Indicated for more accurate FHR or contraction tracing
- May be implemented only after amniotic sac is ruptured
- FHR measured by spiral electrode attached to presenting part
- Uterine tone measured by intrauterine pressure catheter (IUPC)
  - Resting tone of uterus averages 15–20 mm Hg
  - Contraction tone of uterus averages 50–75 mm Hg

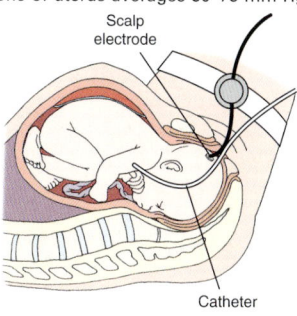

Scalp electrode

Catheter

Internal fetal monitor.

Evaluating Fetal Heart Rate Patterns

- Evaluate FHR baseline
  - Normal baseline FHR is 110–160 bpm
  - Evaluated between contractions over 10 minutes
  - Documented by rounding to nearest 5 bpm
  - Does not include accelerations or decelerations
  - Influences on FHR
    - Central nervous system
      - Fetal sleep ↓ variability of FHR
      - Fetal movement ↑ variability of FHR
    - Autonomic nervous system
      - Sympathetic branch (↑ FHR)
      - Parasympathetic branch (↓ FHR)

- Baroreceptors
  - Respond to ↓ blood pressure with subsequent ↓ FHR
- Chemoreceptors
  - Sense ↓ oxygenation and ↑ FHR
■ Evaluate variability

Variability

■ Fluctuations in FHR baseline over time
■ Important indicator of fetal well-being
■ Sensitive to hypoxia and changes in pH
■ Visually assessed noting peak and trough in beats per minute
  (Expected pattern highlighted in red)

Variability	Possible Cause
Absent (undetectable)	Fetal acidemia
Minimal (≤5 bpm)	Maternal medication Fetal sleep
Moderate (6–25 bpm)	Adequate fetal oxygenation
Marked (>25 bpm)	May be an early sign of mild fetal hypoxia

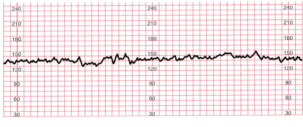

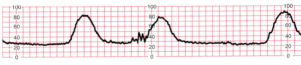

Normal fetal heart rate. (Top, fetal heart rate; Bottom, contractions.)

Tachycardia

- FHR greater than 160 bpm for ≥10 minutes
- Possible cause:
  - Infection/hyperthermia
  - Maternal medications (e.g., terbutaline, albuterol)

Bradycardia

- FHR less than 110 bpm for ≥10 minutes
- Possible cause:
  - Vagal stimulation
  - Interruption of fetal blood flow/gas exchange
  - Maternal medications
- Determine presence of periodic or episodic changes to FHR
  - Periodic: Occurs with uterine contractions
  - Episodic: Not related to uterine contractions

Accelerations

- Sudden increase of fetal heart rate over baseline ≥15 bpm lasting ≥15 seconds
- Indication of fetal well-being
- Etiology: Sympathetic nervous system stimulation

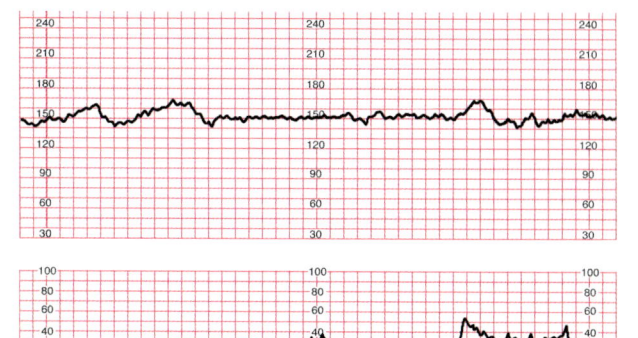

Acceleration. (Top, fetal heart rate; Bottom, contractions.)

Decelerations (Early, Late, Variable)

- Recurrent decelerations: occur with ≥50% of contractions
- Intermittent decelerations: occur with ≤50% of contractions

Early Deceleration

- Decrease in FHR with contractions
- Mirrors the contraction
- **Onset** occurs **before** the contraction peak
- Recovery to baseline rate occurs by contraction end
- Usually benign finding; continue to monitor FHR pattern
- Etiology: Fetal head compression

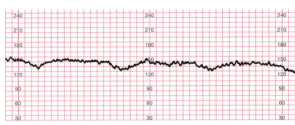

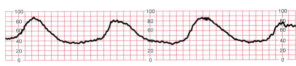

Early deceleration. (Top, fetal heart rate; Bottom, contractions.)

Late Deceleration

- Decrease in FHR occurring with contractions
- **Onset with** or **after** the peak of contraction
- Recovery to baseline rate occurs after contraction ends
- Repetitive pattern
- Etiology: Decreased uteroplacental blood flow/oxygen delivery related to:
  - Hypertension
  - Tachysystole
  - Preeclampsia

- Chronic maternal disease
- Placental decomposition
- Requires intervention

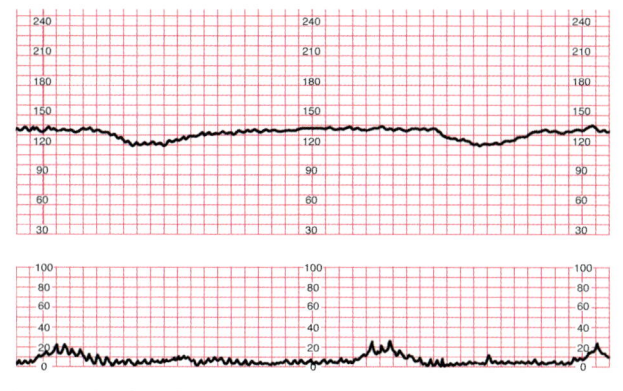

Late deceleration. (Top, fetal heart rate; Bottom, contractions.)

Variable Deceleration
- Decrease in FHR occurring without regard to contractions
- Can range from mild to severe
- May be persistent or occasional
- Shaped like a "V" or "W"
- Onset *variable*
- Variable decelerations that warrant closer monitoring and/or action
    - Repetitive and/or deep decrease in FHR
    - Associated with minimal variability
    - Prolonged with slow return to baseline FHR
- Etiology:
    - Cord prolapse
    - Umbilical cord compression
        - Amnioinfusion may relieve cord compression

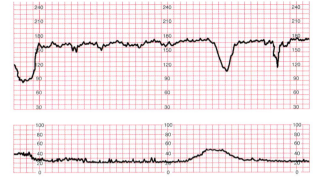

Variable deceleration. (Top, fetal heart rate; Bottom, contractions.)

Nursing Interventions for Intrauterine Resuscitation

- Turn patient to side-lying position
  - Shifts weight of gravid uterus off of the inferior vena cava
  - Allows for improved uteroplacental blood flow
- O_2 via mask at 8–10 L/min
  - Improves oxygen delivery to fetus
- Discontinue IV oxytocin
  - Decreases uterine contractions, thus improving uteroplacental blood flow
- Hydrate patient with IV bolus (500 mL lactated Ringer's [LR])
  - Corrects identified maternal hypotension
- Alter pushing efforts to provide more time for fetal recovery between pushes
- Notify primary health-care provider
- Document nursing interventions, effectiveness of interventions, and orders from primary health-care provider

Monitoring Contractions

Frequency

- Beginning of one contraction to the beginning of the next contraction
- Documented as range, for example, "every 2–5 minutes"
- Tachysystole is defined as >5 contractions in a 10-minute window, averaged over 30 minutes, and should be corrected

Duration

- Beginning of the one contraction to the end of the same contraction
- Documented as a range, for example, "lasting 60–90 seconds"

Intensity

- Palpate uterus both during and after contraction
- Resting tone palpated between contractions
- Document intensity of uterine contractions (findings subjective unless monitored with IUPC)

Intensity	Palpated by Nurse
Mild	Fundus easily indented
Moderate	Requires more pressure to indent fundus
Strong	Unable to indent fundus

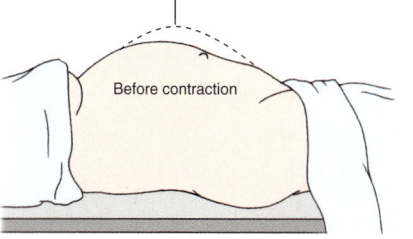

During contraction

Before contraction

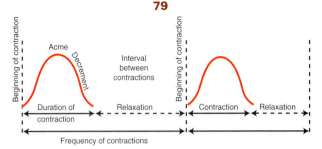

Nursing Care of the Laboring Patient

- First Stage of Labor: Dilation
  - Divided into three phases: Latent, active, transition
- Five Ps of Labor: Nurses should assess and provide interventions to facilitate:
  - Passageway (birth canal)
  - Passenger (fetal attitude, lie, presentation)
  - Powers (contractions)
  - Position (maternal)
  - Psychological response

First Stage of Labor—Dilation

Stage 1—Latent Phase

- **Power:** Contractions palpate mild, every 5–10 minutes, lasting 30–45 seconds
- **Psyche:** Patient is usually excited about the start of labor
- Measuring progress in labor: Cervical dilation (0–3 cm)
- **Passageway:** Encourage frequent position changes that optimize fetal descent, rotation, and widen pelvic outlet
  - Ambulation (with intact amniotic sac)
  - Squatting
  - Hands and knees position
  - Rocking chair
  - Side-lying

- Check bladder status and encourage patient to void every 2 hours
- Provide enema if appropriate/ordered
- Hydration
  - Oral fluids as ordered
  - Monitor intake and output

Nursing Considerations
- Monitor vital signs every 30–60 minutes
- Fetal heart tones every 30–60 minutes

Pain Management
- Pain medication usually avoided until in active labor
- Techniques for pain management
  - Hydrotherapy
    - Shower
    - Labor tub
  - Massage
    - Effleurage
    - Counter-pressure to back
  - Relaxation techniques
    - Progressive relaxation
    - Patterned breathing
    - Soft music and lighting
  - Distraction

Stage 1—Active Phase
- **Power:** Contractions palpate moderate to strong, every 2–5 minutes lasting 40–60 seconds
- **Psyche:** Patient may have greater difficulty coping with the pain of contractions
- Measuring progress in labor: Cervical dilation (4–7 cm)
- **Passageway**
  - Encourage frequent position changes
  - Check bladder status and encourage patient to void every 2 hours

Nursing Considerations
- Monitor vital signs every 30 minutes
- Fetal heart tones every 15–30 minutes

Pain Management
- Continue with effective techniques used in latent phase
- Systemic medications to decrease pain perception
- Document and report maternal and fetal response to medications
- Neonatal side effects related to both dose and timing of administered medication

Systemic Pain Medications in Labor

Medication Class	Drug Action	Nursing Considerations
Opioid agonists • Meperidine (Demerol) • Fentanyl (Sublimaze) **Opioid agonist-antagonist** • Butorphanol (Stadol) • Nalbuphine (Nubain) **Opioid antagonist** • Narcan	↓ Pain perception Reverses opioid-induced respiratory depression	• Side effect: Nausea and vomiting, sedation, dizziness, respiratory depression, transient changes to FHR • Avoid dosing close to delivery to avoid neonatal sedation and respiratory depression • Monitor and report adverse changes to FHR • Causes maternal drowsiness; use safety precautions to prevent falls • Do not give to women who are opiod dependent—may cause abrupt withdrawal
H1-receptor antagonist • Promethazine (Phenergan) • Hydroxyzine (Vistaril) • Diphenhydramine (Benadryl)	↓ Nausea ↓ Anxiety	• Augments opioid analgesics • Monitor and report adverse changes to FHR • Causes maternal drowsiness; use safety precautions to prevent falls
Sedatives	↓ Anxiety Promotes rest in early or prolonged latent phase	• Should not be used in active labor because of potential for prolonged depressant effect on neonate

Stage 1—Transition

■ **Power:** Contractions palpate strong, every 1.5–3 minutes, lasting 45–90 seconds

■ **Psyche:** Patient may feel a loss of control; provide encouragement to patient

■ Measuring progress in labor
  ■ Cervical dilation (8–10 cm)
  ■ Fetal descent (0/+1 station)

- Physical changes common with transition
  - Urge to push if presenting part is low
  - Nausea/vomiting
  - Trembling limbs
  - Beads of sweat on upper lip
  - Increased bloody show
- **Passageway:** Activity more restricted; however, encourage positions that promote fetal rotation and descent
  - Squatting
  - Hands and knees position
  - Side-lying

Nursing Considerations
- Encourage patient to void
- Monitor vital signs and fetal heart tones every 5–15 minutes

Pain Management
- Continue with effective techniques used in active phase
- If systemic medications are given, consider amount of time estimated until birth and potential for newborn effects (respiratory depression)
- Have naloxone hydrochloride (Narcan) available to reverse effects if needed
- Document maternal and fetal response to medications

Second Stage of Labor—Expulsion

- 10 cm dilated until the birth of the baby
- **Power:** Contractions palpate strong, every 2–3 minutes lasting 60–90 seconds
- **Psyche:** Patient may be eager or afraid to push
- Measuring progress in labor
  - Descent of fetus: from +1 station to crowning
    - Cardinal movements of labor
    - Engagement/Descent/Flexion
    - Internal rotation
    - Extension
    - External rotation
    - Expulsion
- **Passageway**
  - Wait for urge to bear down; "Ferguson reflex"
  - Discourage prolonged breath-holding
  - Encourage open glottis pushing

- **Position** for pushing
  - Squatting
  - Side-lying
  - Modified lithotomy
- Encourage patient to void
  - Patient may pass stool with pushing

Nursing Considerations

- Monitor vital signs every 15–30 minutes
- Fetal heart tones every 5–15 minutes

Pain Management per Primary Health-Care Provider

- Pudendal block: Blocks pudendal nerve
  - Anesthetic effect to lower vagina and perineum for vaginal birth; useful with forceps delivery
- Local anesthesia: Numbs perineum for episiotomy/laceration repair

Prepare for the Birth of the Baby

- Cleanse the perineum
- Ensure working order of suction equipment, oxygen, radiant warmer
- Gather and prepare neonatal resuscitation equipment
- Prepare delivery instruments
- Note precise time of birth.

Immediate Care of the Newborn

General Guidelines

- Any resuscitation equipment should be present, prepared, and in working order
- Maternal history, including gestational age and status of amniotic fluid, should be reviewed to anticipate need for resuscitation
- Notify nursery personnel when delivery eminent
- The American Academy of Pediatrics (AAP) and the American Heart Association (AHA) have established Neonatal Resuscitation Guidelines; the nurse should attend required classes and obtain certification; visit www.pediatrics.org for the latest updates on these guidelines

Initial Steps

- Assess **airway** and **breathing effort**
- Place infant on prewarmed radiant warmer in "sniffing" position

- Remove excess secretions from infant's mouth and then nose
- Provide tactile stimulation to infant by drying

Next Steps
- Simultaneously assess respirations, heart rate, color
  - Heart rate should remain >100 bpm
  - Color should be pink (may have acrocyanosis)
  - Breathing with vigorous cry
  - Fetal position flexed with active movement
- Determine need and provide resuscitation efforts per Neonatal Resuscitation Program (NRP) guidelines
- Protect thermal environment
  - Remove wet towels and lay infant on warm blankets
  - Place temperature probe on infant skin
  - Keep temperature of labor room warm
- After infant is stabilized, encourage kangaroo care
- Document Apgar score at 1 and 5 minutes

Apgar Score			
Score	0	1	2
Heart rate	Absent	Low <100	Normal >100
Respiratory effort	Absent	Slow, irregular	Good; crying
Muscle tone	Limp	Some flexion of extremities	Active motion
Reflex irritability	No response	Grimace	Cough, sneeze, or vigorous cry
Color	Blue or pale	Body pink; extremities blue	Completely pink

Score of 10 possible; score of ≥8 desirable

- Assess for abnormalities that may need immediate attention (e.g., neural tube defects, open lesions, or birth injuries)
- Examine umbilical cord and count number of vessels
  - 2 arteries and 1 vein
  - Place plastic clamp on cord

- Identification
  - Fingerprint mother and footprint newborn
  - Apply identification bands to both mother and newborn before leaving birthing room
- Administer medications
  - Administer eye prophylaxis
    - Ophthalmic antibiotic ointment
  - Administer AquaMEPHYTON (vitamin K)
    - Administer IM in the vastus lateralis muscle
    - Boosts production of clotting factors in newborn
- Weigh, measure, and plot findings on growth chart
  - Assess head, chest, and abdominal circumference
  - Assess length
  - Assess skin for lacerations, bruising, or edema
  - Document passage of stool/urine

Third Stage of Labor—Delivery of Placenta

- **Power:** Strong uterine contractions cause the placenta to detach from the uterine wall
- **Psyche:** Patient may be exhausted; encourage bonding with baby
- Signs of placental separation
  - Sudden gush or trickle of blood from vagina
  - Lengthening of visible umbilical cord at introitus
  - Contraction of the uterus
- Nursing considerations
  - Instruct patient to push when appropriate
  - Note time of placenta delivery
- After placenta expelled
  - Monitor amount of bleeding
  - Monitor vital signs
  - Assess fundus
    - Height
    - Location
    - Tone
  - Administer medications to contract uterus as ordered
    - Prevents hemorrhage
      - Oxytocin (Pitocin)
      - Methylergonovine maleate (Methergine)
      - Ergonovine maleate
      - Prostaglandin (Hemabate)

- Cleanse and apply ice pack to the perineum
- Provide clean linen under patient
- Provide warm blanket: Patients often tremble/shiver immediately after the birth
- Assess level of consciousness/comfort
- Place newborn in arm of mother, encouraging skin-to-skin contact
- Assist with positioning for breastfeeding and bonding

Nursing Care With Intrapartum Procedures

Amniotomy

- Artificial rupture of amniotic sac performed by the primary health-care provider during a vaginal examination to augment contraction frequency and intensity
- Nursing care
  - Pad bed to absorb amniotic fluid
  - Assess fetal heart tones before procedure
  - Note color, consistency, odor, and amount of amniotic fluid
  - Document time of amniotomy
  - Document fetal heart tones immediately after amniotomy
  - Document cervical dilation, effacement, station, and fetal presentation
  - If presenting part is not engaged, limit patient activity to prevent cord prolapse
  - After amniotic sac is ruptured, there is potential for infection
    - Monitor maternal temperature every 1–2 hours
    - Limit number of vaginal examinations

Amnioinfusion

Installation of fluid into the uterine cavity
- Decreases occurrence of cord compression associated with low amniotic fluid volume
- Attempt to correct variable decelerations

Before Procedure
- Consent is signed and placed on patient chart
- Warm fluid if fetus is preterm

During Procedure

The nurse assesses:

- Maternal vital signs
- FHR pattern
- Duration and intensity of uterine contractions
- Fundal height changes
- Monitor amount infused and amount returned
- Note color, odor of returning fluid

REPORT complications:

- Signs of infection
- Maternal or FHR changes
- Increased uterine tone
- Lack of fluid return

Cervical Ripening

- Facilitates cervical softening, effacement, and dilation
- Indicated when there is a medical need for induction of labor and cervix unfavorable
- Methods:
  - Laminaria tents (mechanical cervical dilator made from seaweed)
  - Prostaglandin E1-misoprostol (Cytotec)
  - Prostaglandin E2-dinoprostone (Cervidil Insert, Prepidil Gel)
- Nursing care
  - Monitor FHR and contraction status for 20–30 minutes before procedure
  - Encourage patient to void before insertion
  - Position side-lying position after procedure
    - Monitor maternal vital signs, contractions, and fetal status frequently (per hospital protocol)
    - Report adverse reactions to physician
      - Tachysystole
      - Category II or III FHR patterns
      - Nausea, vomiting, diarrhea
    - Assess pain and provide comfort measures
    - Ensure proper waiting period between cervical ripening and oxytocin administration

Cesarean Birth

- Indications for cesarean birth
  - Cephalopelvic disproportion (CPD)
  - Malpresentations
  - Placenta previa/abruption
  - Umbilical cord prolapse
  - Fetal intolerance to labor
  - Maternal medical conditions
- Preoperative care
  - Place signed consent on chart
  - Insert urinary catheter
  - Remove contact lenses, nail polish, jewelry, prosthetic device, dentures
  - Position wedge under right hip
- Perform preoperative teaching
- Assist significant other to prepare for observation of surgery
- Notify newborn nursing team of eminent delivery
- Administer preoperative medications
- Continue to monitor vital signs and FHR
- Postoperative care
  - Assess respiratory/cardiac status/O_2 saturation
  - Encourage patient to turn, cough, and deep breath
  - Assess level of pain and medication needs
  - Monitor intake and output
  - Assess bowel sounds
  - Assess incision
  - Assess effects of anesthesia
  - Monitor vaginal bleeding and provide pericare
  - Assess vital signs and level of consciousness
  - Assess extremities for circulation

Epidurals in Labor

Before Procedure
- Witness consent/place on patient chart
- Gather and assemble oxygen, suction equipment; place emergency medications at bedside
- Document maternal vital signs and FHR
- Document patient mobility, level of consciousness, and pain

- Encourage patient to void
- Administer IV bolus before epidural insertion to prevent maternal hypotension as ordered

During Procedure

- Position and support patient during insertion of epidural catheter
- Note maternal vital signs before and after test dose, then every 5 minutes with administration; thereafter, monitor vital signs and FHR per hospital protocol
- Frequently evaluate bladder status and encourage to void; catheterize if unable to void and bladder distended
- Assess for level of anesthesia and level of consciousness
- Monitor for comfort with contractions
- Monitor progress of labor (contraction status/cervical changes)
- Assist with position changes
- Report adverse effects
  - Hypotension
  - Pruritus (itching)
  - Pyrexia (fever)
  - Respiratory depression

Induction of Labor

- Artificial stimulation of uterine contractions to facilitate vaginal delivery
- Commonly performed in postterm pregnancy
- Before induction of labor, the nurse should note:
  - Indication for induction
  - Gestational age
  - Any contraindications for procedure
  - Bishop's score
    - Assigned by primary health-care provider before induction of labor
    - Higher scores indicate ↑ likelihood of successful labor induction
    - Parameters of Bishop's score
      - Degree of dilation (1–3 points)
      - Percent of effacement (0–3 points)
      - Station (0–2 points)
      - Consistency of cervix (0–2 points)
      - Cervical position (0–2 points)

Oxytocin (Pitocin)

Hormone that stimulates uterine contractions to induce or augment contractions.

- Assess mother and fetus 20–30 minutes before oxytocin administration
- Initiate oxytocin administration
  - Administer IV piggyback per electronic infusion pump
  - Started at small dose and gradually increased until contractions every 2–3 minutes (follow hospital protocol)
- Monitor maternal-fetal tolerance to procedure
  - Uterine resting tone
  - Contraction frequency, duration, and intensity
  - Intake and output
  - Fetal heart tones (baseline, variability, changes)
  - Cervical dilation and effacement
  - Vital signs
  - Patient comfort
- Monitor for complications of oxytocin (may become evident as dosage increases)
  - Tachysystole
  - Category II or III FHR patterns
  - If complications become apparent
    - Change position to lateral side-lying
    - Discontinue IV oxytocin
    - Provide oxygen per mask at 8–10 L/min
    - Increase rate of nonadditive IV solution
    - Call primary health-care provider

Vaginal Birth After Cesarean (VBAC)

Women who have had a previous cesarean birth may be candidates for vaginal birth.

- Previous cesarean uterine incision documented as low transverse
- No contraindications noted to VBAC
- Physician and surgical team readily available for emergent cesarean birth
- Patient and physician agree that VBAC is desirable
- Risks of vaginal birth following cesarean must be explained, including:
  - Uterine rupture with possible loss of fetus or uterus
  - Unsuccessful trial of labor with subsequent cesarean

■ Location of previous uterine scar must be documented

Low Transverse   Low Vertical   Classic

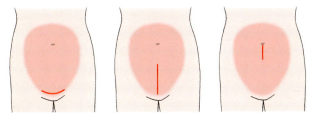

Uterine scars.

Nursing Care

■ Closely monitor uterine response to labor
■ Monitor fetal response to labor
■ Initiate IV access
■ Monitor for signs of uterine rupture
  ■ Severe abdominal pain; "ripping" sensation
  ■ Category II or III FHR patterns
  ■ Cessation of uterine contractions
  ■ Ascending station of presenting part
  ■ Vaginal bleeding
  ■ Signs of maternal shock

Complications in the Intrapartum Period
Prolapsed Umbilical Cord

Umbilical cord slips below/wedges next to presenting part.
■ May lead to fetal hypoxia due to cord compression
■ Possible cause
  ■ Rupture of membranes without engaged presenting part
  ■ Noncephalic fetal presentation
■ Symptoms
  ■ Prolonged variable deceleration
  ■ Pulsating cord palpated upon vaginal examination
  ■ Visible cord at introitus

- Nursing actions
  - Stay with patient and call for assistance
  - Apply sterile glove and hold pressure of presenting part off umbilical cord
  - Place patient in Trendelenburg position
  - Notify physician
  - Monitor fetal heart tones
  - Place sterile saline gauze over any exposed cord
  - Notify obstetrical team; prepare for cesarean birth

Shoulder Dystocia

Difficulty with the fetal shoulder passing under the maternal pubic arch.
- Clinical findings
  - Turtle sign
  - Delay in delivery of shoulders after delivery of head
- Nursing interventions
  - Assess bladder status; catheterize if necessary
  - McRobert's maneuver
  - Suprapubic pressure
  - Change in maternal position
    - Hands-knees
    - Squatting
    - Lateral recumbent
  - After delivery
    - Careful assessment for postpartum hemorrhage
    - Careful assessment for newborn injury

Vaginal Bleeding After 20 Weeks' Gestation

Placenta Previa
Low-lying position of placenta in the uterus that partially or completely covers the cervical os.

Clinical Findings
- Painless, bright red vaginal bleeding
- Bleeding may be reported after intercourse
- Uterine tone soft upon palpation
- Medical intervention dependent on:
  - Amount of bleeding
  - Labor status

- Gestational age
- Fetal response
- If labor is active and os is completely covered, C/S indicated
- If bleeding is controlled and labor absent, conservative management
  - Conservative management teaching
    - Activity limitations
    - No sexual intercourse or tampon use
    - Monitor and report bleeding
    - Patient instructed to report placenta placement when admitted to hospital
    - Cesarean preparation class
    - Count fetal movements

Abruptio Placentae

Premature separation of the placenta; may be partial or complete.

Clinical Findings

- Abdominal pain (sudden onset, intense and localized)
- Fundus firm, boardlike, with little relaxation
- Vaginal bleeding
  - Bleeding may be concealed within the uterine cavity
- Alteration in FHR pattern

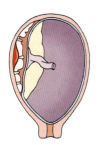 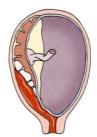 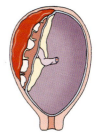

| Partial separation (concealed hemorrhage) | Partial separation (apparent hemorrhage) | Complete separation (concealed hemorrhage) |

Nursing Care With Vaginal Bleeding in Late Pregnancy

- Monitor amount of bleeding
- Check vital signs

- Observe for signs of shock
- Evaluate fetal heart tones
- Palpate uterine tone
- Apply electronic fetal monitor (EFM)
- REPORT category II and III FHR patterns
- REPORT tachysystole
- Do not attempt vaginal examination until placenta placement verified
- Initiate IV fluids
- Report laboratory and ultrasound findings
- Prepare staff for possible cesarean birth
- Attend to patient's emotional needs

Common Postpartum Terms and Abbreviations

Term/Abbreviation	Definition
Afterbirth cramps	Intense uterine contractions that occur in the postpartum period and with nursing; increased intensity with multiparity
Approximation	Closeness of the edges of a healing wound
Colostrum	Thin, yellow breast milk seen in late pregnancy and first 1–3 days postpartum
Coombs', direct	Serum screen for presence of Rh+ antibodies in fetal cord blood
Coombs', indirect	Serum screen for presence of Rh+ antibodies in maternal serum
Dorsal recumbent	Positioning of the patient supine with knees flexed and feet resting on the bed
Endometritis	Inflammation of the uterine lining
Episiotomy	Surgical incision of perineum made to facilitate vaginal birth
Fundus	Upper, rounded portion of the uterus
Homans' sign	Pain in calf upon dorsiflexion of foot
Kangaroo care	Positioning the newborn and mother skin-to-skin with blanket covering both mother and newborn for added warmth
Kegel exercise	Tightening of the perineal muscles performed to strengthen tone
Lochia	Postpartum vaginal discharge consisting of blood, mucus, and tissue
Macrosomia	Newborn with excessive birth weight, usually >4000 gram or >90th percentile for gestational age
Mastitis	Inflammation and infection of the breast
Postpartum	Period of time after childbirth
Sitz bath	Device used to immerse the perineum in warm water that emits a gentle spray to promote healing/comfort

Continued

Common Postpartum Terms and Abbreviations—cont'd

Term/Abbreviation	Definition
Uterine atony	Inability of the uterine muscles to contract after delivery
Uterine involution	Process by which the size of uterus decreases in a predictable pattern

Fourth Stage of Labor

First 1–2 hours after birth.

Immediate Nursing Care

- Assess height, location, and tone of the fundus
- Quantify amount of vaginal bleeding and presence of clots
  - 1 gm = 1 mL blood loss
- Assess condition of the perineum
  - Cleanse and apply ice pack
- Provide clean linen under patient
- Provide warm blanket: Patients often tremble/shiver immediately after the birth
- Assess vital signs
- Assess level of consciousness/comfort
- Encourage bonding of mother and infant using kangaroo care
- Assist with proper latch-on to initiate breastfeeding
- Maintain IV fluids
- Administer uterotonic medication
  - Promote uterine contractions
  - Decrease amount of vaginal blood loss

Nursing Assessment of the Postpartum Patient

- Assess every 15 minutes for the first hour
- Assess every 30 minutes for the second hour

- Assess every 4 hours for the first 24 hours
  - Uterine tone
  - Bleeding
  - Perineum
  - Bladder status
  - Vital signs
    - Blood pressure
    - Pulse
    - Respiration
    - Temperature every 1–4 hours
- Fluid balance
- Circulation to extremities
- Comfort/level of consciousness
- Newborn interaction

Postpartum Assessment and Nursing Care

Remember the acronym BUBBLE-HE.

Breasts
Uterus
Bowel
Bladder
Lochia
Episiotomy
Homans' sign
Emotions

Breast Assessment

- Consistency: Soft, filling, or firm
- Nipple
  - Type: Inverted, flat, or everted
  - Integrity: Bleeding, cracked, intact
  - Redness
  - Comfort
- Breast care for the lactating patient
  - A supportive bra should be worn
  - Breast pads placed inside the bra will absorb leaking milk
  - Soap should not be used on breasts; Montgomery's glands secrete oil to keep nipples supple

- After feedings, leave colostrum/breast milk on nipples and expose the breasts to air
- If separated from newborn, initiate breast pump
- Breast care for the nonlactating patient
  - Supportive bra, breast binder, or sports bra
  - No nipple stimulation
  - Do not express breast milk
  - Ice packs/analgesics for engorgement
- Teach breast awareness

Uterus

- Uterine involution
  - Assess the height, location, and tone of the uterus with the patient dorsal recumbent
  - Uterus returns to nonpregnant state in a predictable pattern
  - Fundal height decreases 1 cm per day in the 1st postpartum week
  - Fundal height is documented in centimeters above or below the umbilicus
  - Location of the fundus should be midline and not deviated to the left or right (suggestive of a full bladder)

Postpartum Period	Level of the Fundus	Document
After birth	At the umbilicus	U/U
12 hours after birth	1 cm above umbilicus	1/U
24 hours after birth	1 cm below the umbilicus	U/1
Day 2	2 cm below the umbilicus	U/2
Day 3	3 cm below the umbilicus	U/3

U = umbilicus

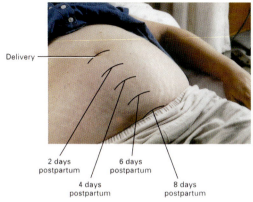

Delivery

2 days postpartum

4 days postpartum

6 days postpartum

8 days postpartum

Uterine involution.

- Tone of the uterus should remain firm, not boggy, in the postpartum period
- If fundus is not firm, perform fundal massage
  - Support the lower uterine segment during massage to prevent inversion of the uterus

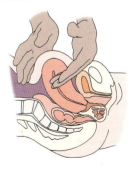

- If fundus is boggy (not firm) after massage
  - Check bladder status and encourage voiding
  - Catheterize (as ordered) if unable to void
- Massage fundus after voiding and note tone and location of fundus
  - Report continued uterine atony to primary health-care provider
- Measures that promote uterine involution
  - Breastfeeding
  - Voiding
  - Fundal massage
  - Uterotonic medications
    - Oxytocin (Pitocin)
    - Methylergonovine (Methergine)
      - If blood pressure elevated, notify primary care provider
    - Carboprost tromethamine (Hemabate)
    - Misoprostol (Cytotec)
    - Dinoprostone (Prostin E2)

Bladder Status

- Postpartum women may have difficulty voiding after birth as a result of the following:
  - Decreased urethral sensation from pressure exerted by the passage of the fetus
  - Side effects of local/epidural anesthesia
  - Delivery trauma to the perineum
- Palpate for bladder distention; bladder should not be palpable above the symphysis pubis
  - A distended bladder will displace the uterus and prevent uterine contractions
  - Catheterization (as ordered) if unable to void or with urinary retention
- Track fluid balance: Intake and output
- Assess for periurethral edema/trauma
- Postpartum diuresis common
  - Rids the body of extracellular fluid
  - Causes the bladder to fill quickly
  - Starts within 12 hours of birth and continues for up to 5 days
  - Urine output may be 3000 mL/day

Bowel

- Auscultate for bowel sounds
- Assess for abdominal distention
- Document bowel movement
- Assess for presence/status of hemorrhoids
  - Encourage the use of sitz baths for comfort
  - Contact primary health-care provider if hemorrhoids present
  - Teach patient how to use prescribed medications
- Educate on prevention of constipation
  - Increase dietary fiber
  - Increase fluid intake
  - Temporary use of stool softeners as prescribed
  - Encourage ambulation

Lochia

Vaginal discharge after delivery is called lochia.
- Blood loss with vaginal birth approximately 500 mL
- Blood loss with cesarean birth approximately 1000 mL
- Note time of last perineal pad change
- Document amount of lochia on perineal pad:
- Weigh blood and clots on perineal pads, under buttocks drapes
- 1 gm = 1 mL of blood loss
- Visual estimation of blood loss is often an underestimation; weighing recommended for improved accuracy
  - Scant (1 inch/2.5 cm mark on pad)
  - Small (<4 inches/10 cm mark on pad)
  - Moderate (<6 inches/15 cm mark on pad)
  - Large (pad saturated ≤1 hour)

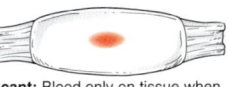

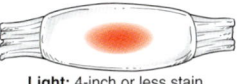

Scant: Blood only on tissue when wiped or 1- to 2-inch stain

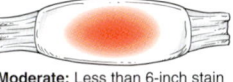

Light: 4-inch or less stain

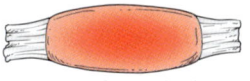

Moderate: Less than 6-inch stain

Heavy: Saturated pad

- Assess the color of lochia; progression of lochia:
  - Lochia rubra (red): days 1–3
  - Lochia serosa (brownish-pink): days 4–9
  - Lochia alba (yellow-white): days 10–14
- Document number and size of blood clots
- Turn patient to assess blood loss under buttocks

Assessment of the Perineum (Episiotomy)

- Use a direct light source to view the perineum
- Position the patient side-lying with top leg forward
- Assess Episiotomy or laceration
  - Redness
  - Edema
  - Ecchymosis
  - Discharge color and consistency
  - Approximated edges

■ Lacerations described by degree of tissue involvement

Degree	Definition
1st	Vaginal mucous membrane and skin of perineum
2nd	Subcutaneous tissue of the perineal body
3rd	Involves fibers of the external rectal sphincter
4th	Through rectal sphincter exposing the lumen of the rectum

■ Avoid enemas or rectal suppositories with 3rd- and 4th-degree lacerations
■ Assess for presence of hematoma; report to primary health-care provider

Extremities (Homans' Sign)

■ Assess circulation to lower extremities
  ■ Pedal pulse
  ■ Color, temperature, blanching
■ Assess for signs of deep vein thrombosis
  ■ Pain
  ■ Swelling
  ■ Redness
  ■ Increased skin temperature
  ■ + Homans' sign
    • Calf pain with dorsiflexion of the foot
■ Prevention of thrombus
  ■ Encourage early ambulation
  ■ Keep legs uncrossed with pressure off the back of knee

Emotional Response

■ Assess interaction with newborn
  ■ Makes eye contact with infant
  ■ Talks to infant
  ■ Holds infant close
  ■ Feeds infant
■ Assess emotional status
  ■ Anxiety
  ■ Crying
  ■ Exhaustion

- Assess for postpartum blues
  - Common occurrence in the immediate postpartum period
  - Period of vacillating emotions
  - Related to physiological changes after birth; intensified with sleep deprivation/postpartum or newborn complications
  - Resolves by 2 weeks postpartum
- Assess for postpartum depression

Vital Signs

Temperature
- Slight ↑ in temperature in first 24 hours common due to dehydration; encourage oral fluids
- If temperature >100.4°F call primary health-care provider

Pulse
- Assess rate, rhythm, and amplitude
- Tachycardia may indicate infection, hypovolemia, or pain

Blood Pressure
- Low blood pressure may indicate orthostatic hypotension or hypovolemia
- Be alert for orthostatic hypotension upon rising
- Dangle at bedside before rising
- Assist with ambulation in immediate postpartum period
- Elevated blood pressure may indicate preeclampsia

Respirations
- Note rate and depth
- Lungs should be clear on auscultation

Level of Comfort

- Ask patient about pain location and intensity
  - Afterbirth cramps
  - Incisional pain
  - Hemorrhoid pain
- Educate patient that postpartum diaphoresis after birth is common (intense sweating that occurs in the early postpartum period ridding the body of excess fluid)

- Effects of epidural anesthesia
  - √ Leg movement/strength
  - √ Presence of numbness and tingling
  - Assist with ambulation

Nutrition

- Assess dietary needs and concerns
- Average weight loss 12 pounds at birth
- Encourage healthy food choices and ample fluids
- Continue prenatal vitamins while lactating and in the postpartum period

Laboratory Data

Compare postpartum laboratory findings to prenatal laboratory test:
- Hemoglobin/hematocrit
- White blood cell count
- Platelet count

The Rh-Negative Patient

- If mother is Rh− √ Rh status of infant
- If infant is Rh+ and maternal antibody status is negative, mother will require injection of Rho(D) immune globulin vaccine within 72 hours of birth

Mother	Infant	Rho(D) Immune Globulin (300 mcg)
Negative	Negative	No treatment needed
Negative	Positive	Administer within 72 hours of birth

Post-Cesarean Birth

- Provide routine postpartum assessment along with following:
    - Effects of anesthesia
    - Level of consciousness
- Ability to hold and care for infant may be limited as a result of the following:
    - Comfort level
    - Limitation in movement
- Respiratory status
    - Pulse oximetry
- Patient-controlled anesthesia (PCA)
    - Determine effectiveness
    - Number of attempts/amount given
    - Side effects
- Abdominal assessment
    - Bowel sounds
    - Abdominal distention
    - Ability to pass flatus
- Incision/dressing
    - Circle drainage and mark with date and time
    - Assess incision with dressing change
        - Approximation
        - Redness
        - Drainage
        - Edema
        - Hematoma
        - Odor
- Nutrition
    - Intake and output
    - Nausea/vomiting
    - Presence of bowel sounds
    - Progression of diet
- Progression of activity
    - Turn/cough/deep breathe
    - Dangle at side of bed
    - Sit up in chair
    - Ambulate with assist

Complications in the Postpartum Period

Postpartum Hemorrhage

Risk Factors
- Uterine and maternal factors
  - Overdistention of the uterus
  - Macrosomia, twins, or polyhydramnios
  - Precipitous labor or prolonged labor
  - Grand parity
  - Chorioamnionitis
  - Maternal obesity
- Placental factors
  - Placenta abruptio
  - Placenta previa
  - Placenta accreta, increta, percreta
- Coagulation deficits
  - Thrombocytopenia
  - Anemia
  - Von Willebrand disease

Etiology
- Uterine atony
- Retained placental fragments
- Vaginal/cervical laceration
- Perineal hematoma

Clinical Findings
- Perineal pad saturated in <1 hour, with or without clots
- Continuous trickle of vaginal bleeding
- Firm, bruised area on perineum
- Tachycardia
- Hypotension
- Decreased O_2 saturation <95%
- Decreased urine output

Interventions
- Identify and correct source of bleeding
- Provide fundal massage until firm while supporting the uterus
- Quantify blood loss
  - Weigh blood-saturated pads

- Check bladder status and monitor urine output
  - Catheterize if needed
  - Report low urine output
- Increase mainline intravenous fluids as ordered
- Administer uterotonic medication as ordered
  - Oxytocin (Pitocin)
  - Methylergonovine maleate (Methergine)
    - If blood pressure elevated, call primary care provider
  - Carboprost tromethamine (Hemabate)
  - Dinoprostone (Prostin E2)
  - Misoprostol (Cytotec)
- Closely monitor vital signs and level of consciousness
- Monitor for signs of hypovolemic shock
  - ↑ Pulse ↓ blood pressure
  - Restlessness
  - Pale, clammy skin
  - Syncope
- Monitor and maintain oxygenation
  - Assess O_2 saturation
  - Administer oxygen as ordered
- Order and report laboratory findings
  - Type and cross-match
  - Complete blood count (CBC), disseminated intravascular coagulation (DIC) profile, comprehensive metabolic profile
- Stay with patient
  - Team member to call primary health-care provider
  - Notify surgical team as needed

Infection

Infections common in the postpartum patient:
- Endometritis
- Wound infection
- Urinary tract infection
- Mastitis

Nursing Considerations
- Encourage frequent hand washing of patient and staff
- Ensure thorough cleaning of equipment
- Obtain cultures as appropriate

- Report abnormal laboratory findings and vital signs
  - Temperature elevation >100.4°F
  - ↑ White blood cell count
- Administer antibiotic therapy as ordered
  - Consider medication safety for lactating patients
- Teach patient signs and symptoms of infection

Endometritis (Infection of the Uterus)
Risk Factors
- Operative birth
- Prolonged labor
- Internal monitoring
- Premature rupture of membranes
- Manual removal of placenta

Clinical Findings
- Enlarged uterus, tender to palpation
- Foul-smelling vaginal discharge .
- Elevated temperature
- Lower abdominal cramping

Mastitis (Infection of the Breast)
Risk Factors
- Alteration in nipple integrity with entry of pathogen
- May be due to improper latch (review technique with patient)
- Delayed emptying of breast milk

Clinical Findings
- Unilateral breast pain, warmth and redness
- Malaise and flu-like symptoms
- Elevated temperature/chills

Nursing Considerations
- If antibiotics compatible, continue with breastfeeding
- Increase rest and fluid intake
- Analgesics, cool packs may help with breast discomfort

Wound infection
Risk Factors
- Operative delivery
- Laceration
- Episiotomy

Clinical Findings
- Incision not well approximated
- Incision red with purulent drainage
- Pain and heat to incision site
- Elevated temperature

Urinary Tract Infection
Contributing Factors
- Catheterization of bladder
- Retention of urine in bladder

Clinical Findings
- Dysuria
- Frequency of urination
- Flank pain

Nursing Considerations
- Teach patient to wipe from the front to back after urination
- Change perineal pads with each void
- Encourage oral fluids
- Encourage foods that ↑ acidity of urine (cranberry juice)

Postpartum Depression

Risk Factors
- History of depression or anxiety disorder
- Prenatal depression
- Inadequate social or partner support
- Large number of life stressors
- May occur 2 weeks postpartum to 12 months after birth

Clinical Findings
- Extreme or unswerving sadness
- Compulsive thoughts
- Feelings of inadequacy
- Loss of appetite
- Inability to care for infant and/or self
- Suicidal thoughts

Interventions
- Psychotherapy
- Medications
- Assistance with newborn care

Thrombophlebitis/Deep Vein Thrombosis

Risk Factors
- History of varicosities
- Advanced maternal age
- Obesity
- Long periods of bed rest
- Occupation that requires long periods of standing
- Clotting disorder

Etiology
- Increased clotting factors in postpartum period
- Infection in the vessel lining to which a clot attaches

Clinical Findings
- + Homans' sign
- Affected site warm to touch
- Swelling, redness, and pain to affected leg

Nursing Considerations
- Interventions dependent on severity of findings
- Administer anticoagulants as ordered
- Monitor coagulation profile
- Compression stockings
- Apply warm, moist heat
- Rest
- Observe for symptoms of pulmonary embolism
  - Dyspnea
  - Chest pain
  - Hemoptysis
  - Patient fearful

Postpartum Education

- Education of the postpartum family is an essential role of the postpartum nurse
- New skills should be discussed, demonstrated, and reinforced
- Document education and patient return demonstration of skills

REPORTABLE SYMPTOMS

Teach the patient to report the following signs and symptoms to the primary health-care provider

- **Signs of infection**
  - Elevated temperature
  - Localized redness or pain to either breast
  - Persistent abdominal tenderness
  - Persistent pain to perineum
  - Burning, frequency, or urgency of urination
  - Foul odor to lochia
  - Redness, pain, or discharge at incision
- **Signs of uterine subinvolution**
  - Increased amount of lochia
  - Resumption of bright red color
  - Presence of clots
- **Signs of thrombophlebitis/deep vein thrombosis**
  - Pain, redness, and heat to lower extremities
- **Signs of postpartum depression**
  - Extreme or unswerving sadness
  - Compulsive thoughts
  - Feelings of inadequacy
  - Inability to care for infant and/or self
  - Suicidal thoughts

Breastfeeding

Advantages of Breastfeeding
- Optimal nutrition for infant
- Monetary savings
- Convenience for mother
- Promotes uterine involution
- Immunoglobulins passed to newborn via breast milk
- Protects the infant from infection
- Decreased incidence of infant:
  - Allergies
  - Otitis media
  - Upper respiratory infections

Positioning
- The infant's body should face the breast, with the ear, shoulder, and hip aligned

- Position pillows to support the weight of the infant
- "C-hold" of the mother's breast assists the latch-on
- Encourage frequent nursing (8–12 feedings in 24 hours)
- Demonstrate positioning of infant for increased comfort
    - Mother should vary positions with subsequent feeding
        - Side-lying
        - Football hold
        - Cradle hold

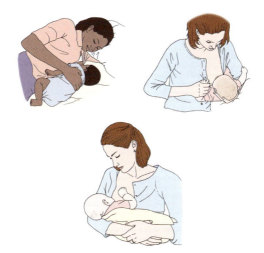

Latch-On

- Proper latch-on is important for maternal comfort, maintaining nipple integrity and the newborn's ability to suckle effectively
- Elicit the rooting reflex by stroking the infant's lower lip
- As the infant's mouth opens wide, bring the infant to the breast, ensuring both the nipple and part of the areola are in the infant's mouth

- Correct latch-on: Infant's jaws will rhythmically move with an audible swallow; mother will express comfort
- Incorrect latch-on: Clicking noise as infant sucks with nipple pain expressed by mother; break suction by placing one finger by the infant's mouth and re-latch

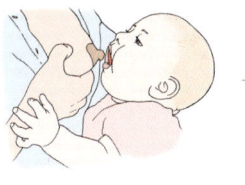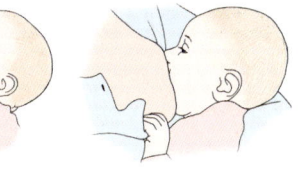

Feeding Schedule
- The newborn should be fed on demand
  - Prolactin releases in response to suckling
  - Stimulates the alveolar cells of the breast to produce the appropriate amount of milk to meet the infant's needs
- The mother should initiate breastfeeding when the infant demonstrates hunger cues
  - Increased alertness or activity
  - Smacking of the lips
  - Suckling motion
  - Moving of the head in search of the breast
- Continue to feed until the infant detaches spontaneously, burp the infant, and continue feeding on the other breast
- Hind milk present later in feeding, rich in fat content
- Start breastfeeding on the breast ended with the last feeding
- Newborns should feed 8 to 12 times per day
- Sleepy newborns should be awakened for feeding by:
  - Changing the diaper
  - Undressing

REPORT breastfeeding concerns to the primary health-care provider:

- Feedings that are consistently short with the infant appearing hungry after feedings and the breasts remaining full
- Swallowing is inaudible once milk is established
- The infant is not gaining the expected amount of weight

- The infant has fewer than six wet diapers a day; urine is amber-colored
- Nipple pain or cracking is present

Engorgement
- Occurs on postpartum day 3–5 as the volume of breast milk ↑
- Subsequent engorgement can be prevented through the following:
  - Frequent feedings
  - Not skipping feedings
- Treatment
  - Express small amount of breast milk manually or with a breast pump so that the breasts will soften and the baby can latch
  - Apply cold packs to breasts intermittently
  - Apply cleaned, cooled cabbage leaves to breasts until warm/wilted
  - Take a warm shower or use warm compress right before feeding

Nutrition
- Add 500 calories more than nonpregnant diet
- Continue prenatal vitamins while lactating
- Stay well hydrated
- Avoid alcohol, smoking, or recreational drugs
- Consult with pediatrician before using any over-the-counter or prescription medication

Pumping and Storing
- Demonstrate use of breast pump
- Store milk in clean glass or hard plastic containers without bisphenol (BPA) in amounts that coincide with newborn intake; plastic bags indicated for breast milk storage should be sturdy and well sealed
- Thaw frozen milk in refrigerator or by running under warm water; do not refreeze
- Write date of expression on storage container and use oldest milk first
- Length of storage dependent on location

Storage Location	Temperature	Guidelines (Optimal Time)
Room temperature	16°–29°C (60°–85°F)	3–4 hours
Refrigerator	4°C (39°F) or lower	72 hours
Freezer	Less than −4°C (24°F)	6 months

Data from Academy of Breastfeeding Medicine Clinical Protocol #8 (2010), Human milk storage information for home use for full-term infants. Breastfeeding Medicine, 5(3), 127–130.

Weaning

- Gradual weaning decreases the likelihood of engorgement
- Remove one feeding at a time
- If infant is younger than 1 year, infant formula, instead of cow's milk, must be given

Breast Care

- Oxytocin release promotes the let-down reflex; moves breast milk forward toward the nipple
  - Causes the uterus to contract producing "afterbirth" pains
  - Can occur when baby cries or with thoughts of the baby
  - Breast pads inside a supportive bra will collect leaking breast milk
- Soap should not be used on breasts; Montgomery's glands secrete oil to keep nipples supple
- After feedings, leave colostrum/breast milk on nipples and expose the breasts to air
- Breast self-examination should be performed after feeding on a chosen day of the month until menses returns
  - Report breast mass, redness, pain, rash, edema, or cracked/painful nipples to primary care provider

Community Resources

Lactation consultant
La Leche League
Primary health-care provider

Uterine/Vaginal Changes

The uterine fundus lowers 1 cm below the umbilicus each day until returning to pelvis on day 10–14.

Normal Progression of Lochia

Lochia progresses from bright red to brown to light pink, also decreasing in amount

REPORT abnormal findings

- Lochia returns to bright red or increases in amount
- Persistent bright red lochia
- Lochia with a foul odor
- Saturating one pad ≤1 hour or passing golf ball–sized clots

Return of the Menstrual Cycle

- Dependent on method of infant feeding
  - If breastfeeding, lactation amenorrhea while exclusively breastfeeding infant (first 6 months)
  - If bottle feeding, menses usually returns 6–8 weeks after delivery
- Remind patient that ovulation returns before menses

Sexuality

- Sexual intercourse may be resumed after lochia has ceased and the episiotomy has healed to prevent infection, trauma, or pain
- Usually recommended after 6-week postpartum checkup
- Vaginal lubrication may be diminished; use water-soluble gel
- Female superior or side-lying position may assist in comfort
- Discuss family planning methods; ovulation returns before menses

Perineal Hygiene

- Stress importance of hand washing before and after perineal care
- Demonstrate use of perineal cleansing bottle
  - Fill bottle with warm water
  - After void, rinse perineum with water
  - Pat area dry from front to back
  - Apply new perineal pad
- Keep perineal pad/underwear from touching floor

Comfort Measures

- Apply perineal ice packs intermittently for the first 24 hours
- Warm water sitz baths may be ordered after 24 hours, usually two or three times a day, for 20 minutes to promote healing and comfort
  - Tighten perineal muscles upon entering sitz bath
- Apply creams, sprays, and ointments to perineum as ordered
- Discuss bowel habits and steps to avoid constipation

Kegel Exercises

Encourage patient to perform Kegel exercises throughout the day to strengthen perineal muscle tone

- To locate muscle, tighten perineal muscles as though stopping the flow of urine (this technique is only used to locate the muscles, not to perform the exercise)
- Hold contraction for several seconds, release, and repeat 10–15 times; discourage breath-holding

Emotions

Postpartum Blues

- Symptoms of postpartum blues include tearfulness, insomnia, and moodiness
- Postpartum blues common in the early postpartum period
- Duration less than 2 weeks
- Possible cause
  - Physical and hormonal changes after birth
  - Exhaustion
- Encourage patient to discuss feelings
- Encourage private time when baby naps
- Discuss the difference between "blues" and depression

REPORT symptoms of postpartum depression

- Extreme or unswerving sadness
- Compulsive thoughts
- Feelings of inadequacy
- Loss of appetite
- Inability to care for infant and/or self
- Suicidal thoughts

Activity Level

- Frequent rest periods will help healing of body and mind
- Patient should nap when baby sleeps
- Avoid lifting anything heavier than the baby
- Limit activities to care of newborn/self
- Ask for assistance with housework/shopping

Common Newborn Terms and Abbreviations

Abbreviation/Term	Definition
Acrocyanosis	Cyanotic appearance of the newborn hands and feet in the immediate newborn period
AGA	Refers to the newborn: **A**ppropriate for **g**estational **a**ge
Babinski's reflex	Elicited by stroking the plantar surface of the newborn foot from heel upward and across the ball to the great toe; expected response: toes fan and hyperextend with dorsiflexion of the great toe
Ballard tool	Physical/neurological assessment of the newborn; used to determine accuracy of gestational age
Barlow's test	Assessment of the newborn hips in which the hip is flexed and the thigh is abducted as it is pushed posteriorly to the line of the femur's shaft; used to detect hip dysplasia
Caput succedaneum	Edematous area on the newborn skull; most often evident on the occiput after vaginal delivery
Cephalohematoma	Unilateral swelling of the newborn head present within the first 3 days of life caused by a collection of blood between the skull bone and the periosteum
Colostrum	Thin, yellow breast milk seen in late pregnancy and first 1–3 days postpartum
Epispadias	Abnormal positioning of the urinary meatus on the dorsal (upper) side of the penis
Erythema toxicum	Newborn rash, often on the face and trunk, characterized by pustules with red base; usually resolves spontaneously
Extrusion reflex	Outward protrusion of the newborn's tongue when touched
Hydrocephalus	Abnormal accumulation of cerebrospinal fluid in the brain

Continued

NEWBORN

Common Newborn Terms and Abbreviations—cont'd

Abbreviation/Term	Definition
Hyperbilirubinemia	Excess of serum bilirubin resulting from breakdown of red blood cells, leading to jaundice
Hypospadias	Abnormal positioning of the urinary meatus on the ventral (under) side of the penis
Imperforate anus	Congenital defect in which the opening to the anus is missing or forms a blind pouch
Kangaroo care	Positioning the newborn and mother skin-to-skin for added warmth
Kernicterus	Deposits of unconjugated bilirubin in brain cells
Lanugo	Downy hair on arms, back, face of the newborn
LGA	**L**arge for **g**estational **a**ge
Mastitis	Inflammation and infection of the breast
Meconium	First newborn bowel movement; greenish-black and tarry
Milia	Small white spots on the newborn nose caused by unopened sebaceous glands; disappear spontaneously
Molding	Elongated shape of the newborn skull resulting from overriding cranial bones to facilitate passage through the birth canal
Mongolian spot	Dark bluish spot that appears most commonly on the buttocks of dark-skinned newborns that gradually fade; may be mistaken for bruise
Moro reflex (startle reflex)	Newborn symmetrically abducts arms with fingers spread to form "C" before returning to flexed position; asymmetrical response may indicate clavicle or brachial plexus injury
Palmer grasp reflex	Newborn fingers curl around examiner's finger when placed in the palm of the newborn's hand

Continued

Common Newborn Terms and Abbreviations—cont'd

Abbreviation/Term	Definition
Plantar grasp reflex	Newborn toes curl downward when examiner's finger is placed at the base of the toes
Polydactyly	Extra digit on hand or foot
RDS	**R**espiratory **d**istress **s**yndrome; due to immaturity of lungs and usually lack of surfactant
Rooting reflex	Newborn's turning of head and opening of the mouth elicited by stroking the lower lip or cheek
SGA	**S**mall for **g**estational **a**ge
Surfactant fluid	Secreted by alveoli of lungs; reduces surface tension of lung fluids, making them more mobile; premature babies often have deficiency
Syndactyly	Webbing between the fingers or toes
Telangiectatic nevi	Flat, deep-pink, easily blanched area of capillary dilation of the skin found on the face or nape of the neck; may fade by second year of life
Tonic neck reflex	Infant's head turned to left, arm/leg on that side extend; same is true when head turned to right
Trunk incurvation reflex	With the infant in prone position, stroke along one side of the spine; infant will curve body toward that side

Nursery Care of the Newborn

- Keep infant warm during all care and procedures
- Assess and record daily weight
- Role-model back positioning
- Keep bulb syringe at bedside
- Check identification bands at each encounter with parents

Physical Assessment of the Newborn

Vital Signs

Reportable findings in red.

- Axillary temperature 97.7°–98.6°F
  - Decreased or increased body temperature (may be a sign of sepsis)
- Auscultate apical pulse for 1 full minute
  - 110–160 beats per minute
  - Sustained resting heart rate below 100 or above 160
- Respirations counted for 1 full minute
  - 30–60 per minute
  - Sustained resting respiratory rate below 30 or above 60

Extremities/Activity

- Newborn posture flexed
- Extremities equal length with full range of spontaneous motion
- Gluteal folds even
- Ten fingers and 10 toes without syndactyly or polydactyly
- Reflexes intact with expected response
  - Moro (startle) reflex: clap your hands loudly or gently bump crib to elicit symmetrical "embrace" movement of infant's arms
  - Babinski: firmly stroke sole of foot to elicit upward movement of great toe and fanning out of other toes
  - Tonic neck: turn infant's face to one side to observe extension of arm on same side and flexion of opposite arm; known as "fencing position"
  - Palmar grasp: place your finger in the infant's palm to elicit curling of his or her fingers around your finger
- Femoral pulse intact and equal in strength/rate compared with brachial pulse
- REPORT:
  - Poor muscle tone or asymmetry of muscle tone
  - Failure to spontaneously move all extremities
  - Decreased range of motion
  - Chewing-like mouth movements combined with noticeable changes in eye and/or body movements (may represent neonatal seizures)

- Unequal knee height, leg length, or asymmetrical gluteal folds (suggestive of hip dysplasia)
- Unexpected response when testing reflexes
- Jitteriness of the extremities (may indicate conditions such as hypoglycemia, hypocalcemia, or drug withdrawal or may be a transient idiopathic finding)

Skin

- Color uniformly pink
- Normal variations
  - Acrocyanosis
  - Milia
  - Lanugo
  - Mongolian spot
  - Telangiectatic nevi "stork bites"
  - Erythema toxicum
- REPORT:
  - Central or circumoral cyanosis (bluish color of mucous membranes mouth; indicates systemic lack of oxygen)
  - Skin lesions, bruises, abrasions
  - Jaundice
    - Routinely assess all newborns for signs of jaundice
      - Blanch skin; if jaundiced, will appear yellow after pressure is released
      - Use bilirubinometer if available
      - Progresses in a cephalocaudal direction (from top to bottom)
    - If jaundice is present, notify primary health-care provider
      - Report serum bilirubin laboratory findings
      - Initiate phototherapy if ordered
      - Have eye shields and diaper in place
      - √ Vital signs, including temperature per hospital protocol
      - Ensure adequate hydration
      - Monitor and report repeat laboratory tests

Head and Neck

- Head round with slight molding or caput succedaneum (soft tissue swelling over large presenting area of skull)

- Anterior and posterior fontanels soft and flat (bulging fontanel normal with crying)
    - Anterior fontanel is diamond-shaped
    - Posterior fontanel is triangle-shaped
- Head held midline with ease of movement
- Trachea midline
- Head circumference > chest circumference
- REPORT:
    - Sunken or bulging fontanels when infant is at rest (bulging fontanel may indicate hydrocephaly; sunken fontanel may indicate dehydration)
    - Cephalhematoma (bulging of head that usually does not cross skull suture line and, because it is filled with blood, is more firm than caput succedaneum)
    - Abrasion
    - Restricted neck movement

Face

- Face symmetrical with rest and crying
- **Eyes** are symmetrical in size and shape; pupils equal; red reflex and corneal reflex intact
- **Nose** is midline with nares patent; √ patency by occluding one nare at a time while assessing breathing
- **Ears** have top of pinna aligned with inner canthus of eyes; pinna well-formed and hearing intact
- **Mouth**
    - Oral mucosa pink and moist; tongue mobile
    - Hard and soft palate intact
    - Strong suck; able to coordinate suck and swallow
    - Tongue freely movable
- Reflexes present
    - Rooting (infant turns head toward side of face that is stimulated)
    - Sucking
    - Gag
    - Extrusion (infant pushes tongue outward when it is touched)
- REPORT:
    - Absence of red reflex
    - Purulent discharge of eyes immediately after birth
    - Low-set ears
    - Lack of response to sound

- Nasal flaring
- Cleft lip or palate
- Large, protruding tongue (possible Down syndrome)
- White patches in mouth (candidiasis)
- Absent rooting, suck, gag, or extrusion reflex
- Severe drooling and/or coughing or gagging (do not feed until condition is assessed)

Chest

- Respirations unlabored
- Chest rises and falls symmetrically
- Lung sounds clear bilaterally
- Clavicles intact
- Breast buds present with nipples prominent and symmetrical
- REPORT:
  - Nasal flaring, chest retractions, or expiratory grunting
  - Asymmetrical or adventitious breath sounds
  - Chest circumference greater than head circumference
  - Loud cardiac murmur with thrill/lift
  - Asymmetrical Moro reflex

Abdomen/Genitals

- Abdomen round and soft without palpable masses
- Three-vessel umbilical cord with drying base
- Bowel sounds present
- First void within 24 hours
  - May be rust-stained from uric acid crystals
- Meconium stool passed within 24 hours
- Female genitalia
  - Labia majora covers minora
  - May have mucoid vaginal discharge or pseudomenses
- Male genitalia
  - Urinary meatus at tip of penis
  - Testes descended with rugae present
- REPORT:
  - Drainage of urine or feces from umbilicus
  - Liver more than 3 cm below right costal margin
  - Abdomen markedly distended
  - Palpable abdominal mass

NEWBORN CARE

- Visible peristaltic waves
- Poor feeding or excessive spitting/vomiting
- Failure to urinate or pass meconium within 24 hours
- Hypospadias or epispadias (urinary meatus on ventral or dorsal side of penis)
- Mass in scrotal or inguinal area
- Imperforate anus

Back

- Spine midline and straight, intact, and easily flexed
- Incurvation reflex intact
- REPORT:
  - Arched back
  - Sinus or nevus with tuft of hair
  - Meningocele/myelomeningocele

Procedures in the Nursery

Blood Sample via Heel Stick

To obtain a blood sample via heel stick:
- Wash hands and apply gloves
- Apply heel warmer to promote vasodilation 5–10 minutes before procedure
- Choose an area on the lateral aspects of the newborn's foot to avoid the median nerve
- Cleanse the skin, use lancet device to puncture skin, obtain sample
- Apply pressure with gauze dressing; after bleeding has stopped, apply bandage
- Provide comfort to the newborn
- Document procedure performed and puncture site

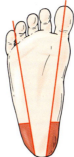

Neonatal Screen

- Blood test performed on the newborn approximately 24 hours after birth, after feeding has been established
- Tests for a variety of genetic and metabolic disorders
- Infants who are discharged early may need to be brought back for newborn screen

Newborn Intramuscular Injection

To perform a newborn intramuscular injection:

- Check written order
  - AquaMEPHYTON (vitamin K)
  - Hepatitis B vaccine
- Obtain parental consent as indicated
- √ Medication is appropriate pediatric dose
- √ Newborn identification
- Choose 25-gauge, ⅝-inch needle
- Choose appropriate site: Vastus lateralis
- Don gloves, cleanse site
- Stabilize the leg; grasp injection site
- Insert needle and administer medication into the vastus lateralis muscle
  - Due to lack of large blood vessels in recommended injections site, aspiration, after needle insertion is not mandatory with immunizations and may increase injection related pain

NEWBORN CARE

- Withdraw needle, apply bandage to site
- Provide comfort to baby
- Document date, time, location, and name and amount of medication
- Assess site for bleeding
- Provide parents with immunization record of vaccines given

Hearing Screen

- Hearing screens are mandated in most states before hospital discharge for early identification of hearing deficits
- Newborns who do not pass the hearing screen should have the screen repeated; referral to audiologist with repeated hearing screen failure
- Report findings to health-care provider/parents

Teaching the Parents of the Newborn

- Education of the postpartum family is an essential role of the postpartum nurse
- New skills should be discussed and demonstrated with appropriate return from parents
- Document education and validate knowledge through verbalization and/or return demonstration
- REPORTABLE SYMPTOMS:
  - Parents should be encouraged to call the pediatrician immediately if they are concerned about their newborn's physical condition or behavior
  - Discharge teaching should include name, phone number, and office address of pediatrician, along with appointment date/time of 1st visit

REPORTABLE SIGNS OF ILLNESS
Parents should be taught to REPORT the following signs to the pediatrician:

- Respiratory distress
  - Nasal flaring
  - Grunting
  - Retractions
  - Rate >60 breaths/minute

- Circumoral cyanosis
- Coughing, choking
- **Abdominal distention**
  - Vomiting, diarrhea, constipation
- **Elevated or decreased temperature**
  - Teach parents how to take an axillary temperature
    - Place thermometer deep into the exposed axilla
    - Gently hold the infant's arm against the chest until digital thermometer beeps
- **Behavior changes**
  - Excessive crying
  - Difficulty arousing
  - Disinterest in feeding
- **Skin changes**
  - Cyanosis
  - Jaundice
  - Rash
  - Redness, swelling, discharge from circumcision site or cord
  - Discharge from eyes
  - Bleeding/discharge/foul odor from cord or circumcision site
- **Signs of dehydration**
  - Sunken fontanels
  - Decrease in number of wet diapers
  - Dry mucous membranes

Normal Newborn Behavior

Pattern of Sleep

- Newborns sleep for short periods; approximately 15–17 hours per day
- Never leave baby unattended on household furniture other than crib
- Reduce the risk for sudden infant death syndrome (SIDS)
  - Back sleeping recommended
  - No smoking around baby
  - Dress baby for comfort; do not overheat
  - Infants should have a close but separate sleeping space
    - Cribs should have slates that are <2⅜ inches apart
    - Choose a firm mattress; should fit snugly in the crib
    - Avoid bumper pads, pillows, stuffed toys, or blankets in the crib

Communication

- Crying is a means of communication and a late sign of hunger
- Teach parents hunger cues
  - Increased alertness or activity
  - Smacking of the lips
  - Suckling motion
  - Moving of the head in search of the breast
- Teach techniques for comforting the fed newborn
  - Swaddling
  - Burping
  - Massage
  - Soft music
  - Diaper change
  - Gentle rocking
- Encourage parents to talk, sing, and hold newborn close
- REPORT:
  - Constant crying
  - Difficulty awakening baby

Newborn Skin Care

Bathing

- Daily bathing of newborns not necessary; keep diaper area clean with each diaper change
- Keep newborn warm by bathing in a warm room free from drafts, keeping bath time short, and wrapping immediately following the bath
- Use only soap recommended for newborn skin with neutral pH
- Stay with baby and hold securely at all times when bathing
- All supplies should be within easy reach
- Test bath water to prevent burns
- No soap is needed on the face
- The eye area should be cleansed with wet cotton balls from the inner to outer canthus
- Dry the baby quickly and cover body to avoid chilling
- Wash hair last to avoid heat loss

Diapering

- After feeding is established expect:
  - ≥6 wet diapers/day
  - Stool that is soft/formed; should not be loose/watery
- Encourage frequent diaper changes
  - Cleanse genital area with mild soap (neutral pH) and water
  - If using disposable wipes, choose those without alcohol or fragrance
  - Cleanse the female genitalia from front to back
  - Do not forcibly retract the foreskin of uncircumcised boys
  - Fanfold diaper to expose umbilical stump to air
- REPORT:
  - Rash or excoriated diaper area
  - Diarrhea/constipation
  - Decreased number of voids

Jaundice

- All newborns should be examined for a yellowish hue to skin and sclera called jaundice
- Jaundice results from elevated bilirubin levels in the newborn
- Requires prompt recognition and treatment to avoid complications, including kernicterus
- Seen initially in the face, progressing to the trunk and extremities
- Promptly REPORT jaundice in newborn skin/eyes so that appropriate laboratory tests and treatment can begin

Umbilical Cord Care

- The cord will fall off spontaneously in 10–14 days
- Do not tug at cord
- Keep area clean, dry, and exposed to air
- Cleanse cord insertion site with water at diaper changes
- Fan fold diaper to expose cord to air
- REPORT redness, drainage, bleeding, foul odor from cord

Circumcision

- Site may be covered with petroleum gauze dressing; tell parents when to remove dressing
- Clean area with warm water for diaper change

- Apply petroleum jelly to head of penis to decrease friction with diaper
- A yellow exudate forms on the head of the penis on day 2–3; this is part of the healing process and removal should not be attempted
- REPORT:
  - Difficulty urinating
  - Persistent bleeding from the site
  - Pus oozing from the site
  - Redness or swelling

Bottle Feeding

Breastfeeding is discussed in the **Postpartum Tab**.

Types of Formula

Directions for dilution of formula on the container must be followed exactly to ensure adequate infant health and nutrition.

Ready-to-Feed Liquid
- Most expensive, but most convenient
- Use without dilution
- Opened cans can be stored in the refrigerator for 48 hours

Liquid Concentrate
- Dilute with equal parts of water
- Prepare enough bottles for the day
- Prepared bottles can be stored in refrigerator for 48 hours

Powdered
- Least expensive
- Add prescribed amount of water for every scoop of powder per manufacturer's instructions
- Shake well to distribute powder

Formula Preparation

- Wash hands
- Clean off can with soap and water before opening
- Mix infant formula with safe water source as defined by local and state health departments
- If concerned about water safety, use bottled nursery water, or If directed, parents can boil tap water for 1 minute and allow to cool completely before mixing with formula
- Prepared bottles can be fed at room temperature

- Refrigerated bottles can be warmed by placing them under warm water to bring to room temperature
- Avoid use of microwave for heating formula

Bottle Preparation

- Bottles should be washed with a brush and soapy water and rinsed thoroughly; nipples can be disinfected by placing in boiling water for 5 minutes and allowed to air dry
- Choose nipples that allow a steady flow of formula but not so large as to cause choking

Technique for Feeding

- Hold close and talk to the infant during feedings
- Parents should avoid propping the bottle (could cause choking)
- Watch baby for hunger cues (usually every 3–4 hours)
  - Increased alertness or activity
  - Smacking of the lips
  - Suckling motion
  - Moving of the head in search of the breast
- Newborns generally drink about 0.5–2 ounces of formula per feeding for the first several days of life
- Elicit the rooting reflex to initiate feeding
- Keep bottle tipped to ensure the nipple remains full of formula
- Burp every 0.5–2 ounces
- The type, amount, and pattern of feedings should be discussed with the pediatrician before hospital discharge
- Formula remaining in the bottle must be discarded
- Demonstrate proper use of bulb syringe in case of choking
- REPORT:
  - Vomiting after feeding
  - Lack of interest in eating
  - Crying after feeding

Safety

- Properly install car seats with belt secured for every trip
  - Infant car seats must be placed in the back seat with the child rear-facing
  - Do not leave child unattended in the car
- Babies should sleep on their backs to decrease the risk for sudden infant death syndrome (SIDS)
- Never microwave a bottle (hot spots may cause burns)

- Protect newborn's skin from excessive sunlight
- Have emergency telephone numbers readily available
- Keep small objects out of reach to prevent choking
- Avoid placing crib near blinds or curtain cords
- Frequently wash hands to prevent spread of infection
- Never leave infant alone on bed, couch, or other elevated surface
- Supervise pets around the newborn
- Be gentle with the baby; DO NOT shake or swing the baby in the air
- Learn infant cardiopulmonary resuscitation (CPR)

Immunizations

- Discuss importance of immunizations for disease prevention
- Provide current schedule of recommended childhood immunizations
- Provide documentation of any immunization given in the hospital

Common Pediatric Terminology and Abbreviations

Term/Abbreviation	Definition
AAP	American Academy of Pediatrics
ABGs	Arterial blood gases; used to measure pH, oxygenation, and carbon dioxide in blood
Abuse	Injurious or potentially injurious treatment of another person; abuse may be verbal, physical, or sexual
Acute abdomen	Sudden severe abdominal pain, in children usually caused by inflammation or obstruction and often requiring surgical intervention
ADD/ADHD	Attention deficit disorder/attention-deficit hyperactive disorder; conditions characterized by distractibility and difficulty focusing attention; ADHD includes excessive motor activity
Adolescence	Period that begins at puberty and lasts until maturity; age is not exact; see definition of puberty
Anemia	Decrease in number or in oxygen binding capacity of red blood cells (RBCs)
AOM	Acute otitis media; middle ear infection caused by bacteria or a virus; common causative organisms are respiratory syncytial virus (RSV), *Streptococcus pneumoniae, Haemophilus influenzae*, and *Moraxella catarrhalis*
ASD	Atrial septal defect; an abnormal opening between the atria of the heart
Asthma	Narrowing and inflammation of airways caused by increased responsiveness
Autosomal dominant	Only one parent must carry the abnormal gene for the child to have the abnormality
Autosomal recessive	Both parents must be carriers of the abnormal gene for the child to have the abnormality

Continued

PEDS
BASICS

Common Pediatric Terminology and Abbreviations—cont'd

Term/Abbreviation	Definition
Bayley	Bayley Scales of Infant Development—standardized tests used to assess development in children ages 2 to 42 mo
BMI	**B**ody **m**ass **i**ndex; a number calculated from measurements of ht and wt • BMI is an indicator of fatness but does not directly measure body fat. In growing children, body fat normally varies according to age and gender; therefore, after calculating a child's BMI, the BMI is compared with a chart that is based on age and gender • **BMI Formula:** Multiply ht in inches by ht in inches then divide the product by wt in lb. Finally, multiply the quotient (answer) by 703. For children, the calculated BMI must be compared with an age- and gender-appropriate CDC chart • For additional information, see http://www.cdc.gov/healthyweight/assessing/bmi/childrens_bmi/about_childrens_bmi.html
BPD	**B**roncho**p**ulmonary **d**ysplasia; inflammation and scarring of the lungs that occurs most often in premature infants, especially in those who have been on mechanical ventilators
BRAT diet	**B**ananas, **r**ice, **a**pplesauce, **t**oast; a diet that is sometimes ordered when a child has diarrhea
Bronchiolitis	Inflammation of bronchioles; most common cause is RSV
Bronchospasm	Spasm resulting in narrowing and partial obstruction of bronchi
Burette	A small fluid volume control container that hangs beneath a larger container of IV fluid; example of brand name is Buretrol

Continued

Common Pediatric Terminology and Abbreviations—cont'd

Term/Abbreviation	Definition
CDC	**C**enters for **D**isease **C**ontrol and Prevention; a federal agency of the Department of Health and Human Services
Celsius or Centigrade (temperature)	Refers to temperature scale. Abbr. = C°; to convert C° to Fahrenheit (F°) multiply degrees in C° by 1.8 and add 32; to convert F° to C° subtract 32 from degrees in F° and multiply by 0.555. For web-based temperature converter tool see: http://www.celsius-fahrenheit.com/
Cephalocaudal	Head-to-toe direction in which development of motor (movement) skills occurs
Colic (infantile)	Characterized by daily or nightly hours of crying. Cause unclear but may be caused by intestinal spasm and pain
Congenital	Present at birth
CP	**C**erebral **p**alsy; damage to motor control center in brain that results in impaired movement and coordination
Cradle cap	Seborrheic dermatitis of the scalp
Critical period	Time during which child is optimally ready for growth or development; failure to progress during this time may impair future growth or development
Croup	Laryngotracheobronchitis; infection-induced (usually viral) inflammation and spasm of the larynx, trachea, and bronchi
Cystic fibrosis (CF)	(Also called mucoviscidosis). Hereditary disease (autosomal recessive) characterized by thick mucus secretions that result in chronic obstructive pulmonary disease (COPD), frequent respiratory infections, pancreatic enzyme deficiency, and poor nutrient absorption. There are abnormal electrolyte concentrations in sweat

Continued

PEDS
BASICS

Common Pediatric Terminology and Abbreviations—cont'd

Term/Abbreviation	Definition
Dehydration	Body deficiency of fluids; in children, it is usually caused by diarrhea and/or vomiting
DDST, DDST-R, DDST II	**D**enver **D**evelopmental **S**creening **T**est *or* **D**enver Developmental Screening Test **R**evised also known as Denver **II**; used to screen for developmental problems in children from birth to 6 years of age; examiners should be trained by an instructor who has been trained by Denver faculty
Development	Growth to maturity; may refer to physical, social and emotional, communicative, or cognitive progress Note that development most often refers to progress in skill and complexity of functioning (see definition of Growth)
Developmental delay	Failure to attain developmental milestones by the expected age
Diarrhea	Passage of unformed stools
Down syndrome	Genetic disorder in which child has 47 rather than 46 chromosomes; mental retardation and other anomalies are common; also known as trisomy 21
Eczema	General term for an itchy red rash that oozes serous fluid and becomes crusty; may be caused by allergy, irritation, drugs, or sun exposure
Emancipated minor	A child who has been granted adult legal status
EMLA	A topical anesthetic
Encephalitis	Inflammation of white and gray matter of the brain; usually caused by a virus and associated with meningitis
Eosinophil	White blood cell (WBC) that is elevated in patient with allergies or parasitic infestation

Continued

Common Pediatric Terminology and Abbreviations—cont'd

Term/Abbreviation	Definition
Epiglottitis	Inflammation of the epiglottis caused by infection; a pediatric emergency that may occlude airway
Erikson	Theorist who proposed eight psychosocial developmental stages from birth to late adulthood (see p 146)
Failure to thrive (FTT)	Weight below 5th percentile on CDC growth charts; may be associated with developmental delays
Fine motor skills	Tasks performed with the small muscles of the hands
Fragile X syndrome	Chromosomal disorder in which there is an abnormality of the X chromosome; a common cause of inherited mental retardation
Freud	Theorist who proposed a psychosexual developmental theory (see p 147)
FOC	**F**rontal-**o**ccipital **c**ircumference; also known as head circumference or HC
FUO	**F**ever of **u**ndetermined **o**rigin
G&D	**G**rowth and **d**evelopment
Gross motor	Tasks performed using large muscles; examples are sitting up, rolling over, walking, lifting
Growth	Usually refers to physical maturation of child
HC	**H**ead **c**ircumference, which is measured at largest circumference
KVO	**K**eep **v**ein **o**pen; abbreviation used to indicate that IV fluids should be delivered as slowly as possible to avoid clotting of the IV needle and line; used when supplemental fluids are not needed but continuous IV access is needed for medication delivery
Lymphocyte	White blood cell (WBC) that increases in viral or chronic infection; normally high in young children

Continued

PEDS
BASICS

Common Pediatric Terminology and Abbreviations—cont'd

Term/Abbreviation	Definition
Maturation	Physical or behavioral change predisposed by genetics and attained by aging and/or environmental influence
Meningitis	Inflammation of covering (meninges) of brain and spinal cord; usually caused by infection
Microdrop	IV drop factor for which 60 gtts equal 1.0 mL of fluid and the rate for mL/hr is the same as the rate of gtts/min (Example: 40 mL/hr = an IV rate of 40 gtts/min)
Mononucleosis (infectious)	Infection caused by Epstein-Barr virus; most common in teens and young adults; also known as the kissing disease
Murmur	Blowing heart sound (similar to a breath sound) • **Functional** murmurs do not indicate heart disease and generally disappear upon return to health; heard in children with conditions such as hypertension • **Innocent** murmurs are caused by vibration associated with increased blood flow such as occurs in a child with fever • **Organic** murmurs are caused by structural changes in the heart or blood vessels
Neonate	Infant in the first 28 days of life
Newborn (NB)	Infant less than 28 days old
N/V/D	**N**ausea, **v**omiting, **d**iarrhea
OME	**O**titis **m**edia with **e**ffusion (also known as serous otitis media [SOM])
ORS	**O**ral **r**ehydration **s**olutions
PDA	**P**atent **d**uctus **a**rteriosus; a congenital condition in which there is failure of the ductus arteriosus to close after birth of the infant; in utero, the ductus arteriosus allows fetal blood to bypass the lungs

Continued

140

Common Pediatric Terminology and Abbreviations—cont'd

Term/Abbreviation	Definition
Percentile	Percentiles on standardized growth charts indicate the percentage of children who are the same age as and who are smaller (wt or ht) or larger than the child being measured, e.g., a child whose ht is plotted on the 45th percentile line of a standardized CDC growth chart is taller than 45% of children of the same age and gender and is shorter than 55% of the same age and gender (CDC charts are based on measurements of a specific group of children and are not globally applicable)
Pertussis	Whooping cough; a disease of the mucous membranes, caused by *Bordetella pertussis*
PKU	**P**henyl**k**eto**nu**ria; congenital autosomal recessive disorder in which there is a failure to metabolize phenylalanine to tyrosine; if untreated, it results in neurological deficits **Phenylalanine** (required for growth and must be obtained from food) is an essential amino acid; amino acids are building blocks of protein and the end product of protein digestion
Piaget	Theorist who proposed stages of cognitive development (see p 147)
PNP	**P**ediatric **n**urse **p**ractitioner; an advanced practice nurse
Preschooler	Period that begins at the end of the toddler stage and ends at school age; usually refers to ages 3 through 6 years
Proximodistal	Center to outward direction in which physical development takes place
Puberty	Stage at which person becomes capable of reproduction; in females, usually between 9 and 16 years of age; in males usually between 13 and 15 years of age

Continued

PEDS
BASICS

Common Pediatric Terminology and Abbreviations—cont'd

Term/Abbreviation	Definition
Reactive airway disease (RAD)	Reversible bronchospasm; asthma
Rheumatic fever	Inflammatory autoimmune condition that may follow untreated or poorly treated group A strep pharyngitis; signs and symptoms include fever, joint pain and redness, uncontrollable movements (Sydenham's chorea), fatigue and painless nodules under the skin; may result in permanent heart damage
Roseola	Viral illness that is most common in infants; usually begins with 3–5 days of high fever followed by a rash
RSV	**R**espiratory **s**yncytial **v**irus; virus that commonly causes cold-like symptoms and may cause serious illness in infants
Rubella	Viral illness that causes rash and fever for 2–3 days; also known as 3-day or German measles; may cause birth defects if acquired by pregnant woman
Rubeola	Measles, which is a viral illness
Scarlet fever	Punctate rash caused by a toxin produced by group A strep; usually follows strep pharyngitis, also known as scarlatina
Shaken baby syndrome	Brain injury cased by shaking baby; brain becomes swollen; bleeding may occur in brain or retina of eyes; may cause permanent damage
Shift to the left	Increased number of immature polysegmented neutrophils, which are WBCs known as stabs or bands; usually increased in acute infection
SOM	**S**erous **o**titis **m**edia; fluid collection in middle ear; common with allergies and after an episode of AOM; also known as OME

Continued

Common Pediatric Terminology and Abbreviations—cont'd

Term/Abbreviation	Definition
Tanner stage	Physical developmental periods based on development of primary and secondary sex characteristics
Tetralogy of Fallot (TOF)	Congenital heart disorder in which there are four congenital abnormalities: 1. Ventricular septal defect (VSD) 2. Pulmonary valve stenosis 3. Right ventricular hypertrophy 4. Overriding aorta—the aorta is positioned over the VSD
Thrush	Candida (yeast) infection of mouth mucosa, most common in children with immunosuppression or in whom antibiotics or corticosteroids are being used
Toddler	Usually child aged 12 to 36 months
Turner syndrome	Chromosomal disorder that affects girls; all or part of one X chromosome is missing; signs are short stature and a webbed neck; other comorbidities are common
Varicella	A viral illness; also known as chickenpox
Viral exanthem	Any of various skin rashes caused by a virus
VSD	**V**entricular **s**eptal **d**efect
X chromosome	Females normally have two X chromosomes, whereas males normally have one X and one Y chromosome

Cultural Competency in Child Health Care

"**Culture**" refers to shared attitudes, beliefs, customs, ideas, language, and moral conduct.

"**Cultural competency**" is indicated by sensitivity to and acceptance of religious, cultural, philosophical, and social preferences of people from

PEDS
BASICS

socioeconomic, ethnic, and/or national backgrounds that are different from one's own. Cultural competence facilitates optimal patient care.

Nursing Actions

Nursing actions that demonstrate cultural competency:
- Respect family dynamics, beliefs, and communication style of different cultures
- Determine beliefs of patients and families regarding illness and appropriate health care
- Avoid criticism of nonharmful folk beliefs or folk remedies
  - When possible, incorporate nonharmful folk remedies into the health-care plan
- Allow all family and support group visits and interactions with the patient that do not jeopardize health care
- Be sensitive to implications of body language and personal space
- Ask permission before touching and examining the child
- Have routine hospital forms and instruction handouts available in languages that are common in the geographical area
- Obtain the services of an interpreter when needed
- Determine whether the family can afford to buy prescribed medications; if not, consult the prescriber to determine whether there is a less expensive alternative or refer for social services support
- Be aware of specific customs and preferences of groups who use the health-care services

Specific Cultural Characteristics

Key Point: Understand common cultural differences, but be aware that there is diversity within cultural groups and that all family members, including children, should be regarded and treated as individuals.

Gender
Some cultures may view gender as a determinate of personal value.
- Arabic and Asian cultures may value a male child more than a female child
- Some cultures believe that the health-care provider should be the same gender as the patient
- Refer to *Interaction With the Health-Care Provider*

Language Barriers

When language is a barrier, patients and families may indicate that they agree with or give consent for whatever is being said to avoid losing face, to prevent social unpleasantry, or to avoid being embarrassed.

- It is very important for some Chinese people to avoid "losing face"

Eye Contact

Eye contact or prolonged eye contact is considered disrespectful in some cultures.

- Vietnamese and some Native American cultures may have specific negative beliefs about eye contact or prolonged eye contact

Body Language

Body language may differ in cultures and may be as important as verbal communication.

- Latinos and other cultures may consider pointing with a finger to be disrespectful; if using a hand signal to indicate that a patient or family should follow you or enter the examination area, use a downward motion of all fingers on one hand rather than holding one finger upward
- Native Americans may consider a prolonged or a firm handshake to be hostile

Response to Pain

Response to pain may differ with culture. Pain may be seen as something to be endured without complaining, or it may be seen as something that should be avoided.

- Native Americans or Vietnamese may believe that pain is to be endured
- Cubans may be very expressive about pain

Beliefs About Illness

- Cultural beliefs may affect the way parents and children view illness
  - Chinese families may view illness as affecting the child's future
- An illness may be believed to have a supernatural origin, such as Voodoo, or it may be believed to be divine punishment
  - Belief of some religious groups and some blacks
  - Navajo Indians may believe that illness represents spiritual and other types of disharmony
- Some cultures fear that strangers may cause supernatural harm to their children
  - Latinos may believe that if a stranger admires a child but does not touch the child, the child may develop "mal ojo" or symptoms of

evil eye, a hex that includes symptoms such as fever, diarrhea, and fussiness
- Illness may also be viewed as an imbalance of "hot and cold" humors (fluids); therefore, each illness is described as "hot" or "cold," and desirable therapies are described as "hot" or "cold." Balance should be restored to the patient by using therapies that are the opposite humor of the disease
  - Belief is common in Latino cultures
- Members of some cultures may carry objects or wear objects around the neck that are believed to guard against witchcraft and/or illness
  - May be important to Native Americans, blacks, and the elderly from various cultures

Interaction With the Health-Care Provider
- Culture may dictate that the parent of one gender or an adult in a particular family position is the person who interacts with the health-care provider
  - In the Hispanic culture, the father is usually the official head of the household and will make decisions regarding treatment of the child
  - In Vietnamese families, the father is the head of the household and interacts with the health-care provider
  - In Native American households, an elder or grandparent may have authority over health-care decisions
- Families from various cultures may consider it disrespectful to question health-care providers

Hospital Visits
Some cultures see office visits or hospitalization as a family affair with a large number of extended family members accompanying the patient to an office visit or to the hospital.
- Important in some Amish religious groups or Romani (Gypsy) families

---

Development Theories

Erikson—Psychosocial Development

In each stage, there is conflict between a psychosocial task and an opposing ego threat.

Stage	Psychosocial Task versus Ego Threat
Birth to 1 year	Trust versus Mistrust
2 to 3 years	Autonomy versus Shame and Doubt
4 to 5 years	Initiative versus Guilt
6 to 12 years	Industry versus Inferiority
13 to 18 years	Identity versus Role Confusion
Young adult	Intimacy versus Isolation
Middle-aged adult	Generativity versus Self Absorption
Elderly adult	Ego Integrity versus Despair

Freud—Psychosexual Development

In each stage, personality conflict may arise as the individual seeks sensual pleasure through a specific body region.

Stage	Description
Birth to 1 year: Oral Stage	Gratification through activities such as sucking, biting, and vocalizing are a major source of pleasure
1 to 3 years: Anal Stage	Activities related to bowel control may affect personality
3 to 6 years: Phallic or Oedipal Stage	The genitals become a focus of attention; penis envy or castration anxiety may occur
6 to 12 years: Latency Period	Further development of previously learned skills occurs
Age 12 years and older: Genital Stage	The genital organs are a major source of pleasure

Piaget—Cognitive (Mental) Development

In each stage, behavior and adaptation to the environment occur through development of intelligence.

PEDS
BASICS

Stage	Description
Sensorimotor Birth to 2 years	Child develops awareness of object permanence; child understands that an object exists even when it has disappeared from view
Preoperational 2 to 7 years	Child is egocentric or unable to see another's point of view
Concrete Operations 7 to 11 years	Child is able to problem-solve by sorting and classifying facts and can think abstractly; reasoning is inductive
Formal Operations 11 to 15 years	Adolescent's thinking becomes more abstract and flexible

Growth/Development Tasks

There is an approximate age range for normal development of each skill. Failure to master a skill at a certain age does not necessarily indicate pathology, but it indicates the need for further assessment and/or referral for further evaluation.

Age	Growth	Skills (Milestones)
0–1 mo	• Ht ↑ 1 in./mo • Wt ↑ 3–5 oz wk • HC ↑ 0.5 in./mo	• Reflex activities—lacks purposeful movement • Lies in flexed position • Regards a person's face
2 mo	• Ht ↑ 1 in./mo • Wt ↑ 3–5 oz wk • HC ↑ 0.5 in./mo	• Lifts head for short periods when prone • Visually tracks moving objects 180 degrees • Smiles and frowns • Coos
3 mo	• Ht ↑ 1 in./mo • Wt ↑ 3–5 oz wk • HC ↑ 0.5 in./mo	• Rolls from back to side • Sits with support • Focuses on own hands • Recognizes parent • Demonstrates pleasure by squealing

Continued

Age	Growth	Skills (Milestones)
4 mo	• Ht ↑ 1 in./mo • Wt ↑ 3–5 oz wk • HC ↑ 0.5 in./mo	• Turns from back to prone position • Holds head erect while in sitting position • Reaches for objects with both hands • Carries objects to mouth • Laughs aloud • Makes consonant sounds
5 mo	• Ht ↑ 1 in./mo • Wt ↑ 3–5 oz wk • HC ↑ 0.5 in./mo	• Turns from abdomen to back • Grasps objects intentionally • Holds object with one hand • Plays with feet
6 mo	• Birth wt has doubled • Ht ↑ 1 in./mo • Wt ↑ 3–5 oz wk • HC ↑ 0.5 in./mo	• Imitates sounds • Stranger anxiety begins
7 mo	Teething begins at 5–7 mos	• Crawls • Bears wt on feet when placed on surface • Transfers object from hand to hand
8 mo	• Ht ↑ 1 in./mo • Wt ↑ 3–5 oz wk	• Sits alone with support • Pulls to standing position • Uses pincer grasp • Marked stranger anxiety • Says "dada" without meaning
9 mo	• Ht ↑ 1 in./mo • Wt ↑ 3–5 oz wk	• Walks while holding on • Bangs 2 blocks together • Drinks from cup • Attempts to feed self • Searches for hidden object
10 mo	• Ht ↑ 1 in./mo • Wt ↑ 3–5 oz wk	• May begin to walk and climb • Neat pincer grasp • Demonstrates one-hand dominance • Plays pat-a-cake and peek-a-boo • May say a few words with meaning

Continued

Age	Growth	Skills (Milestones)
11 mo	• Ht ↑ 1 in./mo • Wt ↑ 3–5 oz/wk	• Cooperates with dressing self • Attempts to feed self with spoon • Can follow one-step commands • Understands meaning of "no" • Shakes head to indicate "no"
12 mo	• Birth wt has tripled • Birth length has increased by 50% • Head and chest circumference are equal	• May walk independently or with hand held • Says "mama" and "dada" with meaning • Points for desired object
15 mo		• Walks unassisted • Pulls or pushes toys • Builds tower of 2 blocks • Scribbles with crayon or pencil
18 mo		• Throws ball overhanded • Builds tower of 3–4 blocks • May be able to control urinary and anal sphincters • Says about 10 words
24 mo	• Weighs about 4 times birth wt • Average wt gain 4–6 lb/yr during years 2–6	• Jumps in place with both feet • Runs with wide stance • Climbs steps by placing both feet on each step • Builds tower of 6–7 blocks • Names familiar objects • Speaks in short phrases
30 mo		• Walks backward • May hop on one foot • Copies a crude circle • Holds crayon with fist

Continued

Age	Growth	Skills (Milestones)
3 yr	All 20 deciduous teeth have erupted	• Rides tricycle • Climbs stairs by alternating feet on steps • Turns doorknobs • Dresses self • Builds tower of 9–10 blocks • Holds crayon with fingers • Copies circle • Speaks in short sentences • Attains bladder and bowel control
4 yr		• Hops on one foot • Recognizes colors • Buttons and unbuttons
5 yr		• Catches ball • Skips and jumps rope • Balances with eyes closed • Sentences contain all parts of speech • Has vocabulary of about 2100 words
6–12 yr	• Ht 2–3 in./yr • Wt 4.5–6.5 lb/yr • Primary teeth are lost and replaced by permanent teeth	• Skips • May learn to swim, ride a bicycle, and roller skate • Learns to read • Language, math, and reasoning skills increase • Peer group becomes increasingly important
12–18 yr	• Continued physical growth • Physical changes of puberty	• Belonging to and acceptance by a group is important • Individual identity and independence are evolving • Sex role identity develops • Thinking is increasingly abstract

Stages of Play

Children normally engage in different types of play during specific periods of development.

- **Solitary play** is the norm before 2 years of age; the child plays alone and resists sharing
- **Parallel play** occurs from ages 2 years until about 5 years; children play along side each other, but without sharing and taking turns with other children
- **Cooperative play** that becomes more organized as the child develops is common in school-aged children; children take turns and enjoy activities that involve participation with other children

Health Promotion/Disease Prevention/Anticipatory Guidance

Infant

Do
- Wash hands before caring for infant
- Begin immunizations as advised by CDC
- Place infant in crib with rails no more than 2⅜ inches apart
- Use a crib mattress that fits snugly in crib to prevent entrapment and suffocation
- Keep crib side rails up when hand is not on infant
- Burp baby during and after feeding
- Place infant on back to sleep
- Cover electrical outlets as soon as baby becomes mobile
- Keep electrical and other cords, such as those on window coverings, out of reach
- Keep small objects out of infant's reach; child explores by putting all objects into mouth
- Keep plants and chemicals out of reach
- Watch siblings and other children when they are near infant
- Use gates at the top and bottom of stairs as soon as infant is mobile
- Use baby monitor system in the home; place monitors in all rooms where infant may be left alone
- Avoid direct sunlight for the first 6 months

- Follow most current age/size car seat guidelines; access online guidelines by typing "CDC car seat safety" into Internet search engine
- Begin tooth brushing with soft brush soon after eruption of first tooth
- Caregivers should be certified in most current guidelines for CPR life support and emergency first aid for children; search for current guidelines online by entering current year followed by "AHA CPR guidelines"
- Recommend that parents attend a newborn/child CPR course
- Keep all available local, state, and national emergency phone numbers (such as police and poison control centers) near the phone or program them into the phone
- Note applicable safety advice for toddlers after infant becomes mobile

Do Not

- Place pillows, stuffed toys, or other objects that might cause suffocation in infant's bed
- Use loose linens that may suffocate or strangle infant
- Use plastic coverings on bedding
- Place crib near window coverings with hanging cords
- Leave crib side rails down while infant is in bed
- Leave infant unattended on changing table or other elevated surface
- Allow infant to hold skin care products while diapers are being changed (products may be ingested, or lids or caps may be swallowed or aspirated)
- Place infant on abdomen (prone) to sleep
- Prop baby's bottle
- Give solid food that may become lodged in airway; hard and/or round foods such as grapes, hotdogs, and nuts pose a risk for choking
- Leave infant alone in bath water
- Leave infant alone in a high chair, swing, or infant seat
- Place infant in the front seat of a car with an airbag
- Use mobile infant walkers that may tip over

Toddler

Do

- Continue immunizations as advised by CDC
- Schedule dental visit by 2½ years of age

- Keep medications, knives, scissors, pins, and needles out of reach or in a locked container; remember that toddlers may climb to reach stored objects
- Remove draw strings from clothing
- Use nonskid backing on area rugs
- Keep furniture and objects with sharp corners out of living area
- Use securely fastened screens in windows
- Turn pot handles toward back of stove
- Keep toilet lid closed when not in use
- Keep guns and ammunition in separate locked areas
- Set temperature of hot water heater to 120°F or lower
- Avoid hanging tablecloths
- Anchor appliances and furniture to prevent them tipping forward onto child who may pull or climb
- Keep doors fastened closed with childproof latches
- Lock pool fences
- Follow most current age/size car seat guidelines; access online guidelines by typing "CDC car seat safety" into Internet search engine
- Talk to children about interactions with strangers
- See Infant Safety for other applicable safety tips

Do Not
- Leave mop water, bathtub water, or other containers of water unattended
- Leave child unattended
- Leave child alone with animals
- Leave windows or outside doors open when child is unattended

Preschooler

Do
- Tell child what to do if lost
- Teach child to call for help and to dial 911
- Consider swimming lessons
- Follow most current age/size car seat guidelines; access online guidelines by typing "CDC car seat safety" into Internet search engine
- Encourage healthy eating habits (see My Plate and Five Food Groups, p 161)
- Encourage regular physical exercise
- Limit screen time (TV, computer, video games) to no more than 2 hours a day

- Encourage all caregivers to set similar and realistic limits on child's behavior
- Plan appropriate disciplinary actions
- See Toddler Safety for other applicable safety tips

Do Not

- Leave child unattended for long periods of time
- Make meal time a battle of wills
- Feed child a diet high in fats and refined carbohydrates

School Age

Do

- Follow most current age/size car seat guidelines; access online guidelines by typing "CDC car seat safety" into Internet search engine
- Encourage healthy eating habits and teach child the basics of nutrition
- Encourage regular physical exercise
- Limit screen time (TV, computer, video games) to no more than 2 hours a day
- Teach pedestrian safety
- Encourage use of bicycle helmet
- Discuss tobacco and substance abuse
- Know and assess for signs of substance abuse
- Discuss normal changes related to sexuality and risk for sexually transmitted infections and pregnancy
- Speak to both child and parent, when appropriate
- Assess for signs and symptoms of depression
- Assess for signs of anorexia and bulimia

Adolescent

Do

- Speak directly to adolescents about their health-care concerns
- Assess sexual practices and safety
- Discuss safe sex and assess need for contraception
- Encourage healthy eating habits
- Assess diet, in particular for anorexia/bulimia as well as for excess fat and/or calorie intake
- Encourage regular physical exercise

- Assess for depression
- Address need for physical exercise
- Discuss and assess for substance use/abuse
- Counsel regarding seat belt use

Nutrition

Breast Milk and Formula

Breast Milk

- American Academy of Pediatrics recommends (2012) breastfeeding for children birth to at least 12 months of age with the addition of complementary foods at about 6 months of age
- Breast milk is easily digestible, so most breastfed infants feed every 2–3 hours

Formula

- Homemade formulas are not recommended
- Regular cow's milk is not recommended for children younger than 12 months of age; this includes canned milk and refrigerated milk
- Commercial infant formulas are used as substitutes for human milk
- Formula-fed infants usually feed every 3–4 hours
- Forms of infant formulas include the following:
  - Liquid, ready-to-use (most expensive of formulas)
  - Liquid, concentrated
  - Powder (least expensive of formulas)
- It is very important to read and follow formula manufacturer's directions carefully; adding water to ready-to-use formula or adding too much water to powder formula or concentrate may cause water intoxication, whereas failure to add enough water to liquid concentrate or powder may lead to diarrhea, dehydration, and kidney failure
- Total formula intake should not exceed 32 oz per day
- Heating formula in a microwave is not recommended, but if a microwave is used, the bottle should be gently shaken, several times, to ensure that the temperature of the milk is even throughout the bottle
- The following table describes uses of infant formulas for infants who are not breastfed; products that are only available for hospitalized neonates are not included

Formulas

(Brand names are subject to changes/additions/deletions. This list includes brand name examples and is not intended to be comprehensive.)

Formula Type and Uses	Formulation Characteristics and Brands
Type: Standard formula **Use:** Normal, healthy, full-term infants	**Characteristics:** • Cow's milk–based • Lactose is the carbohydrate • Contains 20 cal/oz • Butter fat is removed • Vegetable oils and carbohydrates are added • Vitamins, iron, and other nutrients are added **Examples of brands:** • Similac • Enfamil • Good Start • Generic store brands
Type: Extra calories **Uses:** • Premature infants weighing more than 1800 gm • BPD	**Characteristics:** • Cow's milk–based • 22 cal/oz **Examples of brands:** • Enfamil EnfaCare LIPIL (LIPIL is Enfamil's formulation of DHA and ARA) • DHA and ARA are long-chain fatty acids that may be beneficial to premature infants; they are found in breast milk and are thought to be needed for optimal brain and eye development • Similac NeoSure DHA and ARA

Continued

PEDS BASICS

Formulas—cont'd

Formula Type and Uses	Formulation Characteristics and Brands
Type: Soy formula **Uses:** • Milk allergy • Galactosemia • Lactose intolerance (lactase deficiency) • Strict vegetarian diet The American Academy of Pediatrics does NOT recommend soy formulas for low-birth-weight or preterm infants nor for the prevention of colic	**Characteristics:** • Soy product (most contain no lactose) • Corn syrup and/or sucrose as carbohydrate • 20 cal/oz • Lactose-free • Vitamin D, iron, and other nutrients added **Examples of brands:** • Isomil • ProSobee • Alsoy
Type: Protein hydrolysate or casein hydrolysate • A hydrolysate is a compound that is produced when protein is hydrolyzed or "predigested" and converted to a simpler compound **Uses:** • Allergy to cow's milk protein and soy protein (the immune system does not recognize the predigested protein compound as an allergen) • Colic • Cystic fibrosis (malabsorption) • Short bowel syndrome • Bowel resection • Liver disease • Galactosemia	**Characteristics:** • Contains cow's milk and soy • Predigested protein formula (hydrolyzed casein to reduce the possibility of allergy) • All except Nutramigen contain MCT oil (medium-chain triglycerides), which requires fewer enzymes for intestinal absorption • Useful for patients with cystic fibrosis • Nutramigen does NOT contain MCT oil **Examples of brands:** • Alimentum • Nutramigen LIPIL • Pregestimil LIPIL

Continued

Formulas—cont'd

Formula Type and Uses	Formulation Characteristics and Brands
Type: Lactose-free formula **Uses:** • Lactose intolerance • Galactosemia • Temporary use during recovery from infectious diarrhea or gastroenteritis; may decrease cramps and diarrhea	**Characteristics:** • Cow's milk–based or soy product • Contains corn syrup and/or sucrose as carbohydrate source **Examples of Brands:** • Similac Sensitive • Enfamil Lactofree LIPIL • ProSobee LIPIL
Type: Amino acid elemental based formulas (AABFs) **Uses:** • Treatment of conditions that do not provide 100% free amino acids as the protein source (such as Alimentum and Pregestimil) • Severe allergies to cow's milk protein • Eosinophilia-related GI conditions such as eosinophilic gastroenteritis • Cystic fibrosis	**Characteristics:** • Not derived from a traditional food source but from free amino acids • Maximal nutrient breakdown • Dairy-free, gluten-free, hypoallergenic • Amino acid–based • Enfamil PurAmino advertised to be nutritionally complete until 6 months of age and major source of nutrition through 24 months **Example of brands:** • Elecare • PurAmino • Neocate
Type: Low mineral formula **Uses:** • Impaired renal function • Serum calcium disorders, both hypocalcemia and hypercalcemia due to hyperphosphatemia	**Characteristics:** • Cow's milk based • Mineral levels close to that of breast milk **Example of brands:** • PM 60/40 Low Iron (additional iron should be supplied from other sources, and one or more minerals may need to be supplemented)

Continued

Formulas—cont'd

Formula Type and Uses	Formulation Characteristics and Brands
Type: Phenylalanine-free or low-content **Uses:** Phenylketonuria	**Characteristics:** • Cow's milk–based • Amino acids do not include phenylalanine (or content is low) **Example of brands:** • Lofenalac • Alimentum and Pregestimil are low in phenylalanine
Type: Thickened **Uses:** Gastroesophageal reflux	**Characteristics:** • Nonfat cow's milk–based • Contains rice starch that thickens in stomach acid **Example of brands:** • Enfamil A.R. LIPIL
Type: Short-term use **Uses:** Shortens the duration of diarrhea	**Characteristics:** • Milk-free • Lactose-free **Examples of brands:** • Isomil DF

Introduction of Solid Foods

■ Solid foods are not recommended before 4–6 months of age
■ Allow at least 2–3 days between introductions of new foods so that sensitivity to particular foods can be determined
■ Traditionally, iron-fortified infant cereal is the first solid that is offered; after that, fruits and vegetables are added. Some pediatricians suggest that waiting until after 1 year of age to offer eggs and meats may decrease the risk for developing food allergy; however, according to the AAP, there is no solid evidence that offering these foods as early as 4–6 months increases the risk for food allergies
■ Feed solids with a small, rounded spoon, not by adding food to a bottle

- Honey should be avoided because it has been associated with botulism
- Avoid or limit juices because high sugar content may cause diarrhea and add excessive calories to intake
- Well toddlers with normal growth and development may be given whole commercial cow's milk or special toddler formulas
- Toddlers should not be given low-fat milk because the fat in whole milk is needed for brain development
- Children who do not need special diets should have diets based on the recommendations from The United States Department of Agriculture Food and Nutrition Service MyPlate. Related 2015 recommendations and printable resources may be accessed at http://www.choosemyplate.gov/ and at http://www.fns.usda.gov/tn/myplate

THE FIVE FOOD GROUPS

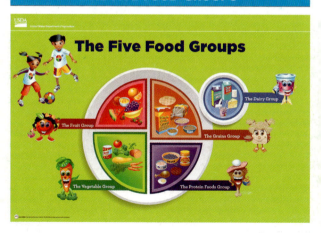

Childhood Immunizations

- Always check the CDC Web site for immunization schedule updates. For links to up-to-date CDC recommendations for childhood immunizations and state guidelines, visit: http://www.cdc.gov/vaccines/ Type "immunizations" into Search bar
- Remember the slogan: "Never miss an opportunity to immunize." This may mean administering immunizations to afebrile children who are in the clinic for episodic health-care visits

Common Conversions

To Convert This	To This	Do This
Centigrade or C°	Fahrenheit or F°	Multiply degrees in C° by 1.8 and add 32
Centimeters (cm)	Millimeters (mm)	Multiply by 10
Centimeters (cm)	Inches (in)	Multiply by 0.394
Cups (c)	Milliliters (mL)	Multiply by 240
Fahrenheit or F°	Centigrade or C°	Subtract 32 from degrees in F° and multiply by 0.555
Milliliters (mL) of IV fluid per hour	Drops (gtts) per minutes	Milliliters per hour is the same as gtts per minute only when using a microdrop set with a drop factor of 60
Inches (in)	Centimeters (cm)	Divide by 2.54
Pounds	Kilograms	Multiply by 0.454
Kilograms (kg)	Pounds (lb)	Multiply by 2.2
Kilograms (kg)	Grams (g or gm)	Multiply by 1000
Grams (g or gm)	Milligrams	Multiply by 1000
Pounds (lb)	Grams (g or gm)	Multiply by .454
Milliliters (mL)	Teaspoons (tsp)	Divide by 5
Liters (L)	Milliliters	Multiply by 1000

Normal Pediatric Lab Values

Test	Range
	Note: Normal values may vary from one laboratory to another and depend on specific test
Arterial Blood Gases	
PaO_2 • Newborn • Child $PaCO_2$ • Newborn • Child	 60–90 mm Hg 75–100 mm Hg 27–40 mm Hg 35–45 mm Hg
pH • 1 day old • Child	 7.29–7.45 7.35–7.45
BUN • Newborn • Child	 3–19 6–18
Calcium • Newborn • Child	 7.6–11.3 mg/dL 8.8–10.1 mg/dL
Chloride	95–107 mg/dL
Erythrocyte Sedimentation Rate (ESR or sed rate) • Child	 Up to 10 mm/h
Hematocrit and Hemoglobin	
HCT • Newborn • Child	 42%–70% 35%–41%
HGB • Newborn • Child	 13–33 g/dL 11.0–16.0 g/dL

Continued

PEDS
BASICS

Normal Pediatric Lab Values—cont'd

Test	Range
Lipids	
• Total cholesterol	Less than 170 mg/dL
• HDL	Greater than 45 mg/dL
• LDL	Less than 110 mg/dL
• Triglycerides	Less than 150 mg/dL
Platelets	150,000–450,000/mm^3
Potassium (K+)	
• Infant	4.1–5.3 mEq/L
• Child	3.4–4.7 mEq/L
RBC	
• Newborn	Up to 7.1 million/mm^3
• Child	4.2–6.2 million/mm^3
Sodium	
• Infant	134–150 mEq/L^3
• Child	135–145 mEq/L^3
Thyroid-Stimulating Hormone (TSH)	Below 10 mIU/L
WBC	
• Newborn	9,000–30,000
• 6 mo old	6,000–16,000
• 1–10 yr old	5,000–13,000
WBC differential	
• Neutrophils (aka granulocytes, PMNs, polys or segs)	54%–75% (lower up to age 2 yr)
• Bands (stabs)	0–5%
• Eosinophils	1%–4%
• Basophils	0–1%
• Lymphocytes	25%–40% (higher up to age 2 yr)
• Monocytes	2%–8%

Well Child Assessment

Note: These physical examination techniques and findings generally apply to young children. Children older than 12 years can usually be assessed according to adult standards.

General Guidelines for Communication With and Assessment of a Child

Allow parent or caregiver to stay in the room; parents may be asked to leave the room during portions of health assessment of the adolescent.

Subjective Data (Questions)
- Sit at the child's eye level when talking to the child or parent
- Assess health history including immunization history and allergies
  - Include prenatal and birth history with APGAR
- Assess family history
- Assess social history; include the following:
  - Relationships with friends and family
  - Home type and people and pets in household
  - Preschool or school achievement
  - Development milestones achieved
  - Sleep habits
  - Behavior problems
  - Type of discipline used and child's response
  - Usual type and amount of exercise
  - Screen time (amount of time spent watching TV or using a computer or playing video games)
  - Diet
  - Substance use/abuse
  - Vehicle restraint use
- Perform review of systems (subjective data related to each body system); speak directly to the child if age appropriate

Objective Data (Physical Examination)
- Approach the child near eye level; sit when possible
- Examine child in the parent's lap if necessary
- Speak in soft, calm voice
- Explain procedures
- Allow the parent or child to remove clothing when necessary
- Weigh children who are younger than 1 year without clothing or diaper

PEDS ASSESS

- Allow the child to handle safe equipment such as otoscope
- Consider demonstrating techniques on a doll
- Use play when possible; example: "open your mouth like a big lion"
- Allow choices when possible—do not offer choices when there are none
- Assessment does NOT need to be in "head-to-toe" order. Perform invasive, embarrassing, or potentially painful procedures last
  - Example: Otoscopic examination of ears, examination of pharynx, or genital examination can be performed at the end of the assessment
- Praise the child for efforts

Assessments and Findings	
Assessment Type and Technique(s)	**Findings**
Listed techniques are used if age appropriate	Normal or expected findings are in black Abnormal findings and possible associated conditions are in red
General	

Assess vital signs	• Vital signs within normal limits for age and gender
	• See Heart and Respiratory Rate for Age Category table on p 185
	• See Blood Pressure for Age and Gender on pp 187–194
	  • Elevated temperature may indicate an internal cause such as infection or may be caused by environmental heat such as sitting or riding in an unairconditioned car during hot weather
	  • Subnormal temperature may be due to illness or environment; note that newborns commonly have subnormal temperatures in response to infection or sepsis
	  • Elevation or decrease of other vital signs may indicate organ malfunction or may occur in response to fever or hypothermia

Continued

Assessments and Findings—cont'd

Assessment Type and Technique(s)	Findings

Neurological

Assess cranial nerves (CNs)	• CNs: Motor and sensory functions intact

Cranial Nerve	Test
I Olfactory	Smell
II Optic	Visual acuity Peripheral vision Color vision Optic disc
III Oculomotor	Six cardinal positions of gaze and pupil constriction
IV Trochlear	Gaze downward and inward
V Trigeminal	Bite down and open mouth Awareness of light touch in mandibular and maxillary area Corneal, also known as "blink" reflex
VI Abducens	Gaze toward temporal side
VII Facial	Smile Make faces Show teeth Identify sweet or salty taste
VIII Acoustic	Hearing Balance
IX Glossopharyngeal	Gag reflex Sour and bitter taste
X Vagus	Gag reflex Uvula Phonation

Continued

PEDS
ASSESS

Assessments and Findings—cont'd

Assessment Type and Technique(s)	Findings
	<table><tr><td>XI Accessory</td><td>Shrug shoulders Turn head side to side</td></tr><tr><td>XII Hypoglossal</td><td>Protrude and move tongue in all directions Push with tongue</td></tr></table> Note that some CNs have both sensory (detect sensation or taste) and motor (movement) functions; when possible, both should be assessed
Assess deep tendon reflexes (DTRs)	• DTRs brisk

Newborns: Assess primitive reflexes such as Moro (startle), tonic neck, rooting, suck, and palmar grasp	• Newborn reflexes within normal limits
	  • Moro reflex limbs form symmetrical embrace when startled
	  • Moro reflex asymmetrical
	• Tonic neck—extends arm and leg on side to which supine infant is turned
	• Roots or searches for nipple when cheek is stroked
	• Grasps finger or object that is placed into hand

Evaluate achievement of developmental milestones	• Age-appropriate developmental milestones attained; see Developmental Milestones on pp 148–151
Evaluate child using the Denver Developmental Screening Test–Revised (DDST-R) or Bayley Scales of Infant Development, if indicated	• Findings within normal limits as determined by testing standards

Continued

Assessments and Findings—cont'd

Assessment Type and Technique(s)	Findings
Skin	
Observe all of skin, including lower back and genital area for children in diapers	• Clean and intact, without lesions or parasites • Redness may indicate infection or burn • Pallor (paleness) may indicate anemia or poor arterial blood supply • Lesions may indicate local or systemic disease • Dimpling or sinus tract at lower spine may indicate underlying spinal disorder or risk for future pilonidal cyst • Scabies is a mite that lives under the skin; it may cause pruritic (itching) punctate lesions on the dorsal side of the finger webs and may cause linear "burrows" under the skin on other parts of the body; in teenagers, scabies may occur in the genital area • Note: A velvety dark color of skin in the axilla or on the back of the neck (acanthosis nigracans) may indicate insulin resistance and that further assessment is needed

Skin Lesion Table

Name of Skin Lesion	Description	Common Causes
Cyst	Elevated mass with palpable borders; contains liquid or semi-solid material	• Cystic acne • Sebaceous cyst
Fissure	Linear break in skin	• Cheilitis • Athlete's foot
Papule	Elevated; palpable	• Raised mole • Insect bite

Continued

PEDS ASSESS

Assessments and Findings—cont'd

Assessment Type and Technique(s)	Findings

Skin Lesion Table—cont'd

Name of Skin Lesion	Description	Common Causes
Macule	Flat; nonpalpable	• Mongolian spot • Port wine stain • Freckle
Vesicle	Fluid filled; size less than 1 cm	• Small blister • Contact dermatitis
Bullae	Serous fluid filled; size greater than 1 cm	• Blister
Pustule	Pus filled	• Acne vulgaris • Impetigo
Plaque	Elevated lesion with rough, flat top, size less than 1 cm	• Psoriasis • Seborrheic keratosis
Nodule	Solid mass; size less than 2 cm	• Lipoma

Nails

Observe color and capillary refill	• Nail beds pink; capillary refill brisk after blanching • Pale nail beds may indicate anemia or response to cold stimuli • Bluish nail beds indicate cyanosis • Slow capillary refill indicates decreased peripheral circulation (due to pathology or cold)

Continued

Assessments and Findings—cont'd

Assessment Type and Technique(s)	Findings
Observe angle of nail attachment to finger	• Base of nail plate forms angle of 130° to 160° at attachment to finger, when viewed from the side • Increase of nail plate angle occurs in clubbing and may indicate chronic respiratory or cardiac problems
Hair	
Observe for infestations	• Clean and free of nits and parasites • Small particles that seem stuck to hair may indicate pediculosis (lice); lice may attach on neck at base of hairline
Observe hair pattern	• Symmetrical distribution of hair with no bald patches on head • Asymmetry of hair distribution or bald areas may indicate hereditary characteristic, abuse, hair pulling, tinea capitis ("ringworm"—not a worm but a fungal infection) that usually manifests as a circular patch of hair loss
Observe hair color	• Hair color is appropriate for race • Unusually pale hair color may indicate albinism • Protein malnutrition may cause brown hair to turn a reddish color
Observe hair texture	• Hair is soft in texture • Coarse or dry hair may indicate hypothyroidism
Head	

Observe head symmetry	• Head symmetrical
	  • During first few days of life, head may be slightly asymmetrical due to molding in infants delivered via vaginal birth
	  • Infants who are placed on their backs to sleep (as recommended) may appear to have flattening of the occiput
	• Marked asymmetry of head

Continued

PEDS
ASSESS

Assessments and Findings—cont'd

Assessment Type and Technique(s)	Findings
Measure head circumference (HC) in children birth to 36 mo of age; measure with a paper tape because cloth tape may be inaccurate due to stretching (See HC growth charts at pp 200–201)	• HC measured at largest circumference; size between 5th and 95th percentile on standardized Centers for Disease Control and Prevention (CDC) growth chart for age and gender • In newborn, HC exceeds chest circumference by 2–3 cm • At 1–2 yr, HC equals chest circumference • In older child, chest circumference exceeds HC by 5–7 cm • HC below 5th may indicate lack of expected brain growth • HC above 95th percentile may indicate hydrocephaly or increased intracranial pressure
Assess fontanels	• Anterior fontanel: 3–4 cm in length, 2–3 cm in width until 9–12 mo of age; closes at 9–18 mo • Posterior fontanel: 0.5–1 cm across; may seem to be closed at birth or by 3 mo of age • Fontanels normally soft and flat; may normally bulge during crying • Abnormally large fontanels or delayed closure may indicate hydrocephaly • Bulging or taunt fontanels in a quiet child may be associated with increased intracranial pressure that occurs with hydrocephaly or meningitis • Premature closure of anterior fontanel may restrict head/brain growth but is sometimes seen in normal children; children with early fontanel closure are monitored closely for abnormal neurological signs
Ears	
Observe placement	• Inner canthus of eyes in alignment with tops of ear pinna; note that outer canthus of eyes may appear higher than top of ears as a result of genetic or racial variation in the slant of the eyes

Continued

Assessments and Findings—cont'd

Assessment Type and Technique(s)	Findings
	• Upper tip of ear pinna located below inner canthus of eye may be associated with intellecutal disability or genetic syndrome

Assess hearing Stand out of child's line of vision and speak or make another sound	• Newborn infant startles to unexpected sound (Moro reflex or startle reflex)
	• Older infant turns head in attempt to localize (find) sound
	• Older child demonstrates intact hearing by repeating or responding appropriately to spoken words or may be assessed using whisper test
	• Failure to respond to sound
	  • Conductive hearing loss
	    • Example is hearing loss caused by cerumen impaction
	  • Sensorineural hearing loss
	    • Example is hearing loss caused by nerve damage or structural abnormalities

Otoscopic examination	• No drainage or foreign body in ear canal
	  • Purulent drainage in ear canal may indicate otitis externa or ruptured tympanic membrane (TM) caused by acute otitis media (AOM)
	  • Impacted cerumen may obstruct hearing and view of TM. Note: Do NOT irrigate ear canals unless the TM is visible and intact
	• TMs and expected bony landmarks visible without redness, retraction, or bulging of TM; redness of TMs is normal in a crying child
	  • Retracted TM and/or air bubbles or air-fluid line behind TM may indicate serous otitis media; also known as otitis media with effusion
	  • Red or bulging TM in quiet child may indicate AOM; viral or bacterial

Continued

Assessments and Findings—cont'd

Assessment Type and Technique(s)	Findings
Eyes	
Observe red reflex	• Red reflex observed bilaterally • Lack of red reflex indicates abnormality in the globe of the eye
Observe corneal light reflex (light reflection in eyes)	• Corneal light reflex is symmetrical; transient asymmetry of corneal light reflex or crossing of eyes may be normal in newborns • Asymmetry of corneal light reflex may indicate strabismus
Observe conjunctiva color and moisture	• Conjunctiva pink without excess tearing • Conjunctival redness (injection) may indicate allergy or infection • Infant: Excess tearing in infant may indicate congenital blocked corneal tear passage (dacryocystitis), irritation, or infection
Assess vision	• **Infant:** Eyes of newborn track bright objects held near face; older infant reaches for toy or has a "social smile" in response to caregiver's smile • **Young child:** Child plays appropriately with toys, observes television without moving close to screen, or names objects on special eye chart with simple recognizable shapes (such as a house or heart) • **Preschooler:** Child identifies direction on a blackbird or Snellen E chart • **School age and older:** Child identifies letters on Snellen chart • Failure to respond appropriately to vision testing should be reported
Nose	
Observe color of mucous membranes	• Mucous membranes pink • Redness of mucous membranes may indicate infection • Paleness may indicate allergy or anemia • Bluish tint may indicate allergy or cyanosis

Continued

Assessments and Findings—cont'd

Assessment Type and Technique(s)	Findings
Observe structure and inspect for lesions inside the nose	• No visible deviated or enlarged structures or polyps • Deviated septum may indicate congenital malformation or history of fracture • Enlarged structures may indicate irritation or infection • Nasal polyps may be associated with allergies, chronic sinusitis, or cystic fibrosis and may result in obstructed nares, mouth breathing, and post-nasal drip
Assess patency of each naris (nostril) by occluding one naris (nostril) at a time	• Child breathes through both nares • Inability to breathe through one naris may indicate congestion or choanal atresia; inability to breathe through both nares usually indicates congestion • Note: Infants are considered to be obligate nose breathers; nasal congestion may compromise oxygenation

Mouth

Observe lips	• Lips moist and free of cracking and fissures • Cracking of lips may indicate mouth breathing due to nasal congestion or air hunger • Fissures in corners of mouth may indicate vitamin deficiency, fungal infection, or irritation
Observe oral mucosa	• Oral mucosa moist, pink, and free of lesions and white plaques • Dry mucosa may indicate dehydration • Red mucosa may indicate irritation or infection (viral or bacterial) • Pale mucosa may indicate anemia or allergy • Mucosal ulcers may indicate autoimmune disorder, stress, viral or bacterial infection • White plaques on mucosa may indicate *Candida* (thrush) infection

Continued

PEDS ASSESS

Assessments and Findings—cont'd

Assessment Type and Technique(s)	Findings
Observe hard and soft oral palates (roof of mouth)	• Hard and soft palates intact without lesions • Cleft (fissure) may congenitally occur in upper lip, hard palate, and/or soft palate of mouth • In infants: Epstein pearls or cysts are benign white or yellow epithelial nodules that occur on the gums or hard palate

Assess dentition (teeth)	• Dentition appropriate for age (see figure on p 209)
	  • Failure of tooth or teeth to erupt
	  • Eruption of permanent tooth before loss of primary tooth
	• No dental caries
	  • Dental caries

Assess position of uvula	• Uvula midline • Slightly deviated uvula may be normal • Deviated uvula may indicate vagus nerve (CN X) lesion or infection including peritonsillar abscess, or may accompany scoliosis
Assess tonsils	Tonsils within tonsillar fossa and pink

Grading of Tonsils

0	Tonsils entirely within tonsillar fossa
1+	Tonsils occupy less than 25% of the area between the anterior tonsillar pillars
2+	Tonsils occupy less than 50% of oropharynx
3+	Tonsils occupy less than 75% of oropharynx
4+	Tonsils occupy 75% or more of oropharynx

• In toddler, tonsils may normally be enlarged but not red or infected

Continued

Assessments and Findings—cont'd

Assessment Type and Technique(s)	Findings

	• In older child, tonsils may be atrophic and appear absent
	   • Red, infected, or enlarged tonsils may impair ability to swallow, which may result in dehydration
	   • Peritonsillar abscess may result in generalized edema and pus collection around one or both tonsils and may impair breathing
	   • Cryptic or scarred tonsils appear to have pits or pockets that may trap food particles or bacteria and may cause chronic sore throat

Assess tongue and frenulum	• Tongue extends over lower gum line • Tongue that does not extend over lower gum line appears "heart" shaped and may indicate ankyloglossia (tongue-tie due to short lingual frenulum)

Neck

Observe for webbing	• No webbing • Webbing of neck may indicate Turner's syndrome
Palpate for lymph nodes Use circular finger motion to palpate nodes	• No palpable lymph nodes • Shotty nodes (*shotty* refers to buckshot or BB-sized nodes) are expected in children; they may signify past infection • Nodes 1 cm or larger; if tender and mobile, often signify infection • Nontender and immobile nodes may signify underlying tumor (attachment to tumor limits mobility) • Unilateral nontender cervical lymph node may signify Kawasaki disease
Palpate thyroid	• No thyromegaly; thyroid may be nonpalpable or detected as a small soft mass on both sides of the trachea • Thyroid mass or enlargement palpable

Continued

Assessments and Findings—cont'd

Assessment Type and Technique(s)	Findings
Assess neck range of motion (ROM)	• Full ROM • Nuchal rigidity demonstrated by limited flexion (chin toward chest) or nuchal rigidity with meningitis • Involuntary muscle contractions manifest as torticollis or wryneck and may be caused by infection or trauma, including birth injury or malpositioning in utero
Auscultate with bell of stethoscope over each carotid artery	• No bruit (pronounced "broo-ee") • Bruit—a blowing sound—indicates arterial obstruction
Cardiovascular	
Observe point of maximum heart impulse (PMI) Observe and palpate for lift and heave (sustained outward thrust of the precordium)	• Point of maximum cardiac impulse (PMI) at the 3rd or 4th intercostal space (depending on age) at the left midclavicular line • No lift or heave • Lift or heave may indicate heart failure
Inspect lips and nail beds for color and capillary refill	• Lips and nail beds pink with brisk capillary refill of nails • Newborns may normally have cyanosis of extremities; called *acrocyanosis* • Central cyanosis (lips) may indicate cardiac or respiratory problem
Assess for peripheral and facial edema	• No edema • Edema may indicate heart failure or fluid overload; facial edema may indicate renal disorder

Continued

178

Assessments and Findings—cont'd

Assessment Type and Technique(s)	Findings
Palpate over precordium for thrill	• No thrill (palpable vibratory sensation caused by a heart murmur) • A thrill indicates that a heart murmur is at least a grade IV–VI
Palpate peripheral pulses bilaterally and simultaneously	• Pulses strong and equal (see illustration of peripheral pulse locations on p 195) • Decreased amplitude of femoral pulses may indicate coarctation of the aorta

Auscultate heart over aortic, pulmonic, tricuspid, and mitral areas	• Heart rate within normal limits for age; see Heart and Respiratory Rate by Age Category table on p 185
	• Regular rhythm
	  • Heart rate may vary markedly as respiratory rate changes (known as *sinus arrhythmia*)
	  • Audible splitting of S_1 and S_2 is common in young children and those with thin chest walls
	• No murmurs
	  • Febrile or anemic children may have transient murmurs
	    • Note whether murmurs are systolic or diastolic
	    • Murmurs are graded on a I–VI scale according to intensity (volume)
	    • Note for murmurs:
	      – Location: Aortic, pulmonic, tricuspid, or mitral area
	      – Radiation: Location of sound
	      – Timing: Early, mid, or late systole or diastole
	      – Character: Crescendo—gradual increase in volume; decrescendo—gradual decrease in volume
	      – Quality: Harsh, blowing, or rumbling
	      – Pitch: High, medium, or low
	      – Variance: With position change or respirations

Continued

PEDS ASSESS

Assessments and Findings—cont'd

Assessment Type and Technique(s)	Findings

Murmur Grade	Description
I	Barely audible
II	Faint but easily heard
III	Soft to moderately loud without palpable thrill
IV	Moderate to loud with thrill (Note that murmur must be at least grade IV to cause a thrill)
V	Loud with thrill; heard with stethoscope partly off the chest
VI	Loud with thrill; heard with stethoscope off chest

Assessment Type and Technique(s)	Findings
Assess blood pressure Use cuff that is at least ⅔ as wide as the upper arm	• Blood pressure between 5th and 95th percentile for height, age, and gender; see table pp 187–194 • Elevated blood pressure in children is most often due to a renal disorder or to obesity • To be accurately diagnosed with hypertension, a child must have systolic or diastolic blood pressure equal to or greater than the 95th percentile on three separate occasions

Respiratory/Chest

Observe shape of chest	• Anterior-posterior (AP)–lateral view of a young child's chest appears rounded; as child grows, the AP–lateral view is about 2:3 • Chest may remain rounded (barrel shaped) in child with chronic respiratory disease such as chronic obstructive pulmonary disease (COPD)

Continued

Assessments and Findings—cont'd

Assessment Type and Technique(s)	Findings
Observe and listen to child's breathing	• Respiratory rate regular and unlabored; rate varies by age: see Heart and Respiratory Rate by Age Category table on p 185 • Periodic breathing (apnea up to 20 seconds is normal in newborns) • Infants and young children are abdominal breathers
Auscultate lungs, all lobes—right middle lobe is auscultated in the right axilla Auscultate all anterior and posterior lung fields	• **Bronchial sounds** are loud and high-pitched hollow sounds that are heard over the upper anterior chest • **Bronchovesicular sounds** are softer tubular sounds heard in the anterior central chest and between the scapula in the posterior chest • **Vesicular sounds** are soft blowing sounds heard throughout peripheral lung fields • Adventitious sounds heard with auscultation may indicate foreign body or mucus in airway, bronchiolitis, asthma, pneumonia, or other pathology • Rales have a crackling sound and are common in pneumonia • Rhonchi are coarse sounds that often clear with coughing • Wheezing, musical, or sibilant rales are whistling sounds that are common with asthma and bronchiolitis
Abdomen	
Observe abdomen	• Abdomen is slightly rounded • Young children are abdominal breathers; abdomen is expected to move with respiratory effort • No visible peristalsis
Palpate abdomen	• No masses or bulges • Young children with a palpable abdominal mass should be assessed for tumor, including Wilms' tumor, a tumor of the kidney • Visible peristalsis may indicate bowel obstruction

Continued

PEDS
ASSESS

Assessments and Findings—cont'd

Assessment Type and Technique(s)	Findings
	• A reducible transient umbilical hernia may exist in infants and young children; most resolve without treatment as muscles strengthen • Nonreducible hernia (report immediately because blood supply may be impaired) • The lower edge of liver may be palpated and percussed about 1–3 cm below the right costal margin (RCM) • Liver that is more than 3 cm below the RCM may indicate heart failure • The tip of the spleen may be palpated and percussed below the left costal margin (LCM) • Palpation of a large area of the spleen may accompany sickle cell disease or infectious mononucleosis
Musculoskeletal	
Assess extremities for symmetry in form, movement, and strength	• All structures are symmetrical in form, movement, and strength; one foot, hand, ear, etc. may normally be slightly larger than the other • Marked asymmetry of structures, movement, or strength may be due to congenital malformation or injury
Assess length or stature and weight and compare with CDC growth charts	• Length (measured supine) or stature (height measured standing) between the 5th and 95th percentile for age and gender (CDC growth charts availability p 197) • Weight between the 5th and 95th percentile for age and gender • Weight or length/stature measurements that are below the 5th percentile or above the 95th percentile on CDC growth charts require further assessment

Continued

Assessments and Findings—cont'd

Assessment Type and Technique(s)	Findings
Observe body mass index (BMI) if 2 years of age or older and compare to charts	• BMI between 5th and 84th percentiles for age and gender (see charts on pp 206–207) Children whose BMI for age and gender is at or above the 84th percentile but below the 95th percentile are termed "overweight" • Children whose BMI for age and gender is at or above the 95th percentile are termed "obese"
Observe spine with child bending forward For best view, observe while standing in FRONT of the child	• Spine midline • **Kyphosis:** Exaggerated convex curvature of thoracic spine • **Lordosis:** Exaggerated concave curvature of lumbar spine • **Scoliosis:** Lateral curvature of spine; most frequent in females and during adolescent growth spurt; uneven shoulder height or uneven hip height may indicate scoliosis
Observe upper extremity structure and range of motion	Moves upper extremities symmetrically, through full range of motion
Observe structure of lower extremities	• Genu varum (bowleggedness) is normal until age 2 years • Bowing of one leg or worsening of this variation beyond 2 years of age may indicate rickets or Blount's disease • Genu valgum (knock-knees) is common in preschoolers • Toes point forward and plantar aspect (bottom) of feet touch level surface when standing • Metatarsus adductus or varus (toeing inward or pigeon toes) is normal in young children • Talipes equinovarus (clubfoot): Plantar aspect of foot turns inward and downward and is not flexible

Continued

PEDS
ASSESS

Assessments and Findings—cont'd

Assessment Type and Technique(s)	Findings
Observe lower extremity range of motion	• Scissoring of lower extremities may indicate cerebral palsy • Flatfeet (arches touch floor when standing) are normal in infancy and early childhood; arch develops during childhood • Moves lower extremities symmetrically, through full range of motion • Toe-walking is common in young toddlers
Male Genitalia and Rectal Area	
Observe skin	• Skin intact without lesions • Lesions may indicate diaper dermatitis, candidal infection, or sexually transmitted disease (STD) or infection
Observe placement of urinary meatus	• Urinary meatus located at tip of penis • Hypospadias: Urethral opening is on the ventral or underside of the penis • Epispadias: Urethral opening is on the dorsal or upper side of the penis
Palpate scrotum for testicles	• Testes descended with rugae present • Cryptorchidism: Undescended testicles
Inspect rectal area	• Rectal area clean and free of lesions and protrusions • Caking of fecal matter may indicate neglect of an infant or poor hygiene in an older child • Lesions may indicate sexually transmitted diseases and/or sexual abuse • Protrusion from the rectum may indicate hemorrhoids or prolapsed rectum (prolapsed rectum more common in child with cystic fibrosis)
Female Genitalia and Rectal Area	
Observe genitalia	• Skin intact without lesions • Lesions may indicate diaper dermatitis, candidal infection, or sexually transmitted disease

Continued

Assessments and Findings—cont'd

Assessment Type and Technique(s)	Findings

	• Labia majora covers labia minora and clitoris
	  • Labia majora are poorly developed in premature infants
	  • A prominent clitoris may indicate a chromosomal abnormality
	• Urethral and vaginal orifices patent
	  • Imperforate vaginal hymen should be referred

Inspect rectal area	• Rectal area clean and free of lesions and protrusions • Caking of fecal matter may indicate neglect of an infant or poor hygiene in an older child • Lesions may indicate sexually transmitted diseases and/or sexual abuse • Protrusion from the rectum may indicate hemorrhoids or prolapsed rectum

Heart and Respiratory Rate by Age Category

Age	Sustained Heart Rate*	Sustained Respiratory Rate*
Full-term newborn	100–160 (higher in premature infant)	30–60
Infant	80–120	30–60
Toddler and preschooler	70–110	24–40
School age and adolescents	60–100	15–26

*Rate may increase during periods of illness or stress and rate may decrease in well conditioned athletes.

Blood Pressure Measurement Interpretation in Children

1. Use the standard height charts (WHO and CDC charts on following pages) to determine the height percentile.
2. Measure and record the child's systolic blood pressure (SBP) and diastolic blood pressure (DBP).
3. Use the correct gender table for SBP and DBP (BP tables follow).
4. Find the child's age on the left side of the table. Follow the age row horizontally across the table to the intersection of the line for the height percentile (vertical column).
5. There (at the intersection described in step 4), find the 50th, 90th, 95th, and 99th percentiles for SBP in the left columns and for DBP in the right columns.
   - BP less than the 90th percentile is normal.
   - BP between the 90th and 95th percentiles is prehypertension. In adolescents, BP equal to or exceeding 120/80 mm Hg is prehypertension, even if this figure is less than the 90th percentile.
   - BP greater than the 95th percentile may be hypertension.
6. If the BP is greater than the 90th percentile, the BP should be repeated twice at the same office visit, and an average SBP and DBP should be used.
7. If the BP is greater than the 95th percentile, BP should be staged. If stage 1 (95th percentile to the 99th percentile plus 5 mm Hg), BP measurements should be repeated on 2 more occasions. If hypertension is confirmed, clinical evaluation and laboratory tests should proceed as described in Table 7 of the Fourth Report of the Diagnosis, Evaluation, and Treatment of High Blood Pressure in Children and Adolescents (Web link p 190). If BP is stage 2 (greater than the 99th percentile plus 5 mm Hg), prompt referral should be made for evaluation and therapy. If the patient is symptomatic, immediate referral and treatment are indicated. Medical treatment is outlined in Table 6 of the Fourth Report of the Diagnosis, Evaluation, and Treatment of High Blood Pressure in Children and Adolescents.

Blood Pressure Levels for Boys by Age and Height Percentile

Age (Year)	BP Percentile	Systolic BP (mm Hg) Percentile of Height							Diastolic BP (mm Hg) Percentile of Height						
		5th	10th	25th	50th	75th	90th	95th	5th	10th	25th	50th	75th	90th	95th
1	50th	80	81	83	85	87	88	89	34	35	36	37	38	39	39
	90th	94	95	97	99	100	102	103	49	50	51	52	53	53	54
	95th	98	99	101	103	104	106	106	54	54	55	56	57	58	58
	99th	105	106	108	110	112	113	114	61	62	63	64	65	66	66
2	50th	84	85	87	88	90	92	92	39	40	41	42	43	44	44
	90th	97	99	100	102	104	105	106	54	55	56	57	58	59	59
	95th	101	102	104	106	108	109	110	59	59	60	61	62	63	63
	99th	109	110	111	113	115	117	117	66	67	68	69	70	71	71
3	50th	86	87	89	91	93	94	95	44	44	45	46	47	48	48
	90th	100	101	103	105	107	108	109	59	59	60	61	62	63	63
	95th	104	105	107	109	110	112	113	63	63	64	65	66	67	67
	99th	111	112	114	116	118	119	120	71	71	72	73	74	75	75
4	50th	88	89	91	93	95	96	97	47	48	49	50	51	51	52
	90th	102	103	105	107	109	110	111	62	63	64	65	66	66	67
	95th	106	107	109	111	112	114	115	66	67	68	69	70	71	71
	99th	113	114	116	118	120	121	122	74	75	76	77	78	78	79
5	50th	90	91	93	95	96	98	98	50	51	52	53	54	55	55
	90th	104	105	106	108	110	111	112	65	66	67	68	69	69	70
	95th	108	109	110	112	114	115	116	69	70	71	72	73	74	74
	99th	115	116	118	120	121	123	123	77	78	79	80	81	81	82

Blood Pressure Levels for Boys by Age and Height Percentile (Continued)

Age (Year)	BP Percentile	Systolic BP (mm Hg) Percentile of Height							Diastolic BP (mm Hg) Percentile of Height						
		5th	10th	25th	50th	75th	90th	95th	5th	10th	25th	50th	75th	90th	95th
6	50th	91	92	94	96	97	99	100	53	53	54	55	56	57	57
	90th	105	106	108	110	111	113	113	68	68	69	70	71	72	72
	95th	109	110	112	114	115	117	117	72	72	73	74	75	76	76
	99th	116	117	119	121	123	124	125	80	80	81	82	83	84	84
7	50th	92	94	95	97	99	100	101	55	55	56	57	58	59	59
	90th	106	107	109	111	113	114	115	70	70	71	72	73	74	74
	95th	110	111	113	115	117	118	119	74	74	75	76	77	78	78
	99th	117	118	120	122	124	125	126	82	82	83	84	85	86	86
8	50th	94	95	97	99	100	102	102	56	57	58	59	60	61	61
	90th	107	109	110	112	114	115	116	71	72	72	73	74	75	76
	95th	111	112	114	116	118	119	120	75	76	77	78	79	79	80
	99th	119	120	122	123	125	127	127	83	84	85	86	87	87	88
9	50th	95	96	98	100	102	103	104	57	58	59	60	61	61	62
	90th	109	110	112	114	115	117	118	72	73	74	75	76	76	77
	95th	113	114	116	118	119	121	121	76	77	78	79	80	81	81
	99th	120	121	123	125	127	128	129	84	85	86	87	88	88	89
10	50th	97	98	100	102	103	105	106	58	59	60	61	61	62	63
	90th	111	112	114	115	117	119	119	73	73	74	75	76	77	78
	95th	115	116	117	119	121	122	123	77	78	78	80	81	81	82
	99th	122	123	125	127	128	130	130	85	86	86	88	88	89	90

Blood Pressure Levels for Boys by Age and Height Percentile (Continued)

Age (Year)	BP Percentile	Systolic BP (mm Hg) — Percentile of Height							Diastolic BP (mm Hg) — Percentile of Height						
		5th	10th	25th	50th	75th	90th	95th	5th	10th	25th	50th	75th	90th	95th
11	50th	99	100	102	104	105	107	107	59	59	60	61	62	63	63
	90th	113	114	115	117	119	120	121	74	74	75	76	77	78	78
	95th	117	118	119	121	123	124	125	78	78	79	80	81	82	82
	99th	124	125	127	129	130	132	132	86	86	87	88	89	90	90
12	50th	101	102	104	106	108	109	110	59	60	61	62	63	63	64
	90th	115	116	118	120	121	123	123	74	75	75	76	77	78	79
	95th	119	120	122	123	125	127	127	78	79	80	81	82	82	83
	99th	126	127	129	131	133	134	135	86	87	88	89	90	90	91
13	50th	104	105	106	108	110	111	112	60	60	61	62	63	64	64
	90th	117	118	120	122	124	125	126	75	75	76	77	78	79	79
	95th	121	122	124	126	128	129	130	79	79	80	81	82	83	83
	99th	128	130	131	133	135	136	137	87	87	88	89	90	91	91
14	50th	106	107	109	111	113	114	115	60	61	62	63	64	65	65
	90th	120	121	123	125	126	128	128	75	76	77	78	79	79	80
	95th	124	125	127	128	130	132	132	80	80	81	82	83	84	84
	99th	131	132	134	136	138	139	140	87	88	89	90	91	92	92
15	50th	109	110	112	113	115	117	117	61	62	64	64	65	66	66
	90th	122	124	125	127	129	130	131	76	77	79	79	80	80	81
	95th	126	127	129	131	133	134	135	81	81	83	83	84	85	85
	99th	134	135	136	138	140	142	142	88	89	91	91	92	93	93

Blood Pressure Levels for Boys by Age and Height Percentile (Continued)

Age (Year)	BP Percentile	Systolic BP (mm Hg) Percentile of Height							Diastolic BP (mm Hg) Percentile of Height						
		5th	10th	25th	50th	75th	90th	95th	5th	10th	25th	50th	75th	90th	95th
16	50th	111	112	114	116	118	119	120	63	63	64	65	66	67	67
	90th	125	126	128	130	131	133	134	78	78	79	80	81	82	82
	95th	129	130	132	134	135	137	137	82	83	83	84	85	86	87
	99th	136	137	139	141	143	144	145	90	90	91	92	93	94	94
17	50th	114	115	116	118	120	121	122	65	66	66	67	68	69	70
	90th	127	128	130	132	134	135	136	80	80	81	82	83	84	84
	95th	131	132	134	136	138	139	140	84	85	86	87	87	88	89
	99th	139	140	141	143	145	146	147	92	93	93	94	95	96	97

BP, blood pressure

* The 90th percentile is 1.28 SD, 95th percentile is 1.645 SD, and the 99th percentile is 2.326 SD over the mean.

Source: Adapted from Department of Health and Human Services, National Heart Lung and Blood Institute, The Fourth Report on the Diagnosis, Evaluation, and Treatment of High Blood Pressure in Children and Adolescents: https://www.nhlbi.nih.gov/files/docs/resources/heart/hbp_ped.pdf.

Blood Pressure Levels for Girls by Age and Height Percentile

Age (Year)	BP Percentile	Systolic BP (mm Hg) — Percentile of Height							Diastolic BP (mm Hg) — Percentile of Height						
		5th	10th	25th	50th	75th	90th	95th	5th	10th	25th	50th	75th	90th	95th
1	50th	83	84	85	86	88	89	90	38	39	39	40	41	41	42
	90th	97	97	98	100	101	102	103	52	53	53	54	55	55	56
	95th	100	101	102	104	105	106	107	56	57	57	58	59	59	60
	99th	108	108	109	111	112	113	114	64	64	65	65	66	67	67
2	50th	85	85	87	88	89	91	91	43	44	44	45	46	46	47
	90th	98	99	100	101	103	104	105	57	58	58	59	60	61	61
	95th	102	103	104	105	107	108	109	61	62	62	63	64	65	65
	99th	109	110	111	112	114	115	116	69	69	70	70	71	72	72
3	50th	86	87	88	89	91	92	93	47	48	48	49	50	50	51
	90th	100	100	102	103	104	106	106	61	62	62	63	64	64	65
	95th	104	104	105	107	108	109	110	65	66	66	67	68	68	69
	99th	111	111	113	114	115	116	117	73	73	74	74	75	76	76
4	50th	88	88	90	91	92	94	94	50	50	51	52	52	53	54
	90th	101	102	103	104	106	107	108	64	64	65	66	67	67	68
	95th	105	106	107	108	110	111	112	68	68	69	70	71	71	72
	99th	112	113	114	115	117	118	119	76	76	76	77	78	79	79
5	50th	89	90	91	93	94	95	96	52	53	53	54	55	55	56
	90th	103	103	105	106	107	109	109	66	67	67	68	69	69	70
	95th	107	107	108	110	111	112	113	70	71	71	72	73	73	74
	99th	114	114	116	117	118	119	120	78	78	79	79	80	81	81

Blood Pressure Levels for Girls by Age and Height Percentile (Continued)

Age (Year)	BP Percentile	Systolic BP (mm Hg) Percentile of Height							Diastolic BP (mm Hg) Percentile of Height						
		5th	10th	25th	50th	75th	90th	95th	5th	10th	25th	50th	75th	90th	95th
6	50th	91	92	93	94	96	97	98	54	54	55	56	56	57	58
	90th	104	105	106	108	109	110	111	68	68	69	70	70	71	72
	95th	108	109	110	111	113	114	115	72	72	73	74	74	75	76
	99th	115	116	117	119	120	121	122	80	80	80	81	82	83	84
7	50th	93	93	95	96	97	99	99	55	56	56	57	58	58	59
	90th	106	107	108	109	111	112	113	69	70	70	71	72	72	73
	95th	110	111	112	113	115	116	116	73	74	74	75	76	76	77
	99th	117	118	119	120	122	123	124	81	81	82	82	83	84	84
8	50th	95	95	96	98	99	100	101	57	57	57	58	59	60	60
	90th	108	109	110	111	113	114	114	71	71	71	72	73	74	74
	95th	112	112	114	115	116	118	118	75	75	75	76	77	78	78
	99th	119	120	121	122	123	125	125	82	82	83	83	84	85	86
9	50th	96	97	98	100	101	102	103	58	58	58	59	60	61	61
	90th	110	110	112	113	114	116	116	72	72	72	73	74	75	75
	95th	114	114	115	117	118	119	120	76	76	76	77	78	79	79
	99th	121	121	123	124	125	127	127	83	83	84	84	85	86	87
10	50th	98	99	100	102	103	104	105	59	59	59	60	61	62	62
	90th	112	112	114	115	116	118	188	73	73	73	74	75	76	76
	95th	116	116	117	109	120	121	122	77	77	77	78	79	80	80
	99th	123	126	125	126	127	129	129	84	84	85	86	86	87	88

Blood Pressure Levels for Girls by Age and Height Percentile (Continued)

Age (Year)	BP Percentile	Systolic BP (mm Hg) Percentile of Height							Diastolic BP (mm Hg) Percentile of Height						
		5th	10th	25th	50th	75th	90th	95th	5th	10th	25th	50th	75th	90th	95th
11	50th	100	101	102	103	105	106	107	60	60	60	61	62	63	63
	90th	114	114	116	118	119	120	121	74	74	74	75	76	77	77
	95th	118	118	119	121	122	123	124	78	78	78	79	80	81	81
	99th	125	125	126	128	129	130	131	85	85	86	87	87	88	89
12	50th	102	103	104	105	107	108	109	61	61	61	62	63	64	64
	90th	116	116	117	119	121	122	123	75	75	75	76	77	78	78
	95th	119	120	121	123	124	125	126	79	79	79	80	81	82	82
	99th	127	127	128	130	132	133	133	86	86	87	88	88	89	90
13	50th	104	105	106	107	109	110	110	62	62	62	63	64	65	65
	90th	117	118	119	121	122	123	124	76	76	76	77	78	79	79
	95th	121	122	123	124	126	127	128	80	80	80	81	82	83	83
	99th	128	129	130	132	133	134	135	87	87	88	89	89	90	90
14	50th	106	106	107	109	110	111	112	63	63	63	64	65	66	66
	90th	119	120	121	122	124	125	125	77	77	77	78	79	80	80
	95th	123	123	125	126	127	129	129	81	81	81	82	83	84	84
	99th	128	129	130	132	133	134	135	87	87	88	89	89	90	91
15	50th	107	108	109	110	111	113	113	64	64	64	65	66	67	67
	90th	120	121	122	123	125	126	127	78	78	79	79	80	81	81
	95th	124	125	126	127	129	130	131	82	82	82	83	84	85	85
	99th	131	132	133	134	136	137	138	89	89	90	91	92	92	93

Blood Pressure Levels for Girls by Age and Height Percentile (Continued)

Age (Year)	BP Percentile	Systolic BP (mm Hg) Percentile of Height →							Diastolic BP (mm Hg) Percentile of Height →						
		5th	10th	25th	50th	75th	90th	95th	5th	10th	25th	50th	75th	90th	95th
16	50th	108	108	110	111	112	114	114	64	64	65	66	66	67	68
	90th	121	122	123	124	126	127	128	78	78	79	80	81	81	82
	95th	125	126	127	128	130	131	132	82	82	83	84	85	85	86
	99th	132	133	134	135	137	138	139	90	90	90	91	92	93	93
17	50th	108	109	110	111	113	114	115	64	65	65	66	67	67	68
	90th	122	122	123	125	126	127	128	78	79	79	80	82	81	82
	95th	125	126	127	129	130	131	132	82	82	83	84	85	85	86
	99th	133	133	134	136	137	138	139	90	90	91	91	92	93	93

BP, blood pressure

* The 90th percentile is 1.28 SD, 95th percentile is 1.645 SD, and the 99th percentile is 2.326 SD over the mean.

Source: the Department of Health and Human Services, National Heart Lung and Blood Institute, The Fourth Report on the Diagnosis, Evaluation, and Treatment of High Blood Pressure in Children and Adolescents. Retrieved from http://www.nhlbi.nih.gov/files/docs/guidelines/child_tbl.pdf.

Heart Auscultation Areas and Peripheral Pulses

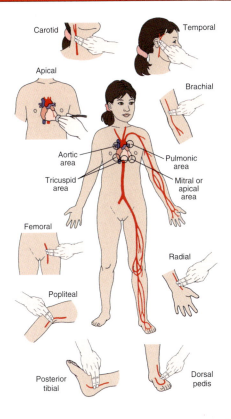

Carotid

Temporal

Apical

Brachial

Aortic area

Pulmonic area

Tricuspid area

Mitral or apical area

Femoral

Radial

Popliteal

Posterior tibial

Dorsal pedis

Lymph Nodes

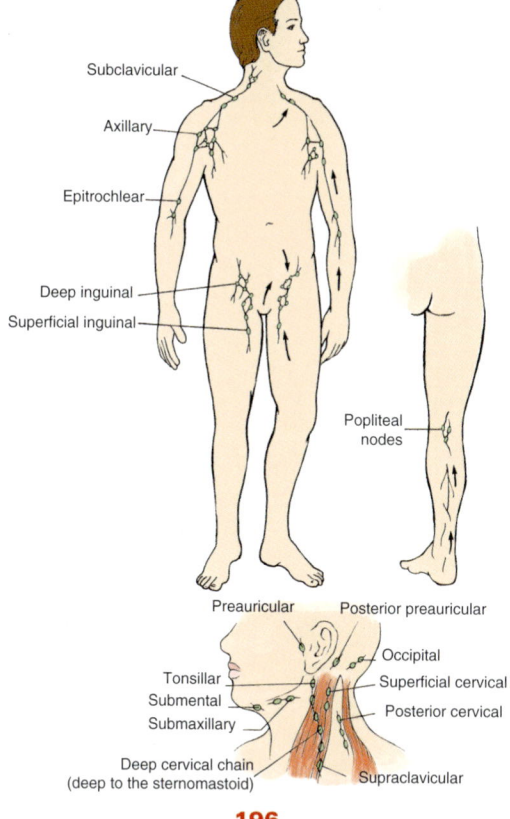

Subclavicular

Axillary

Epitrochlear

Deep inguinal

Superficial inguinal

Popliteal
nodes

Preauricular   Posterior preauricular

Occipital

Tonsillar   Superficial cervical

Submental

Submaxillary   Posterior cervical

Deep cervical chain
(deep to the sternomastoid)   Supraclavicular

Growth Charts

Centers for Disease Control recommends the following:

- World Health Organization (WHO) growth charts be used for infants and children ages 0 to 2 years of age in the United States.
- CDC growth charts be used for children age 2 years and older in the United States.

For training in the use of the growth charts, visit the following Web site: http://www.cdc.gov/nccdphp/dnpao/growthcharts/.

WHO Growth Charts

Use these charts from birth to 2 years of age.

Published by the Centers for Disease Control and Prevention, November 1, 2009. Source: WHO Child Growth Standards (http://www.who.int/childgrowth/en). Retrieved from http://www.cdc.gov/growthcharts/who_charts.htm.

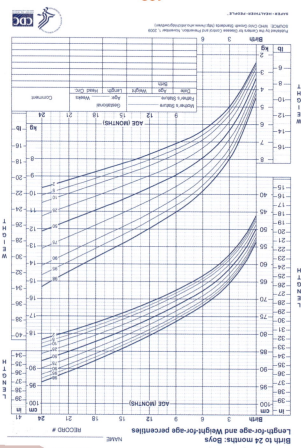

Birth to 24 months: Boys
Length-for-age and Weight-for-age percentiles

NAME

RECORD #

SOURCE: WHO Child Growth Standards (http://www.who.int/childgrowth/en)
Published by the Centers for Disease Control and Prevention, November 1, 2009

Birth to 24 months: Girls
Length-for-age and Weight-for-age percentiles

NAME _____

RECORD # _____

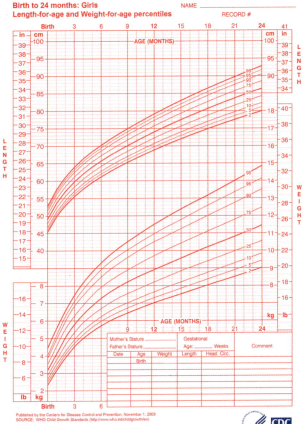

PEDS
ASSESS

Birth to 24 months: Boys
Head circumference-for-age and
Weight-for-length percentiles

NAME

RECORD #

SOURCE: WHO Child Growth Standards (http://www.who.int/childgrowth/en)
Published by the Centers for Disease Control and Prevention, November 1, 2009

201

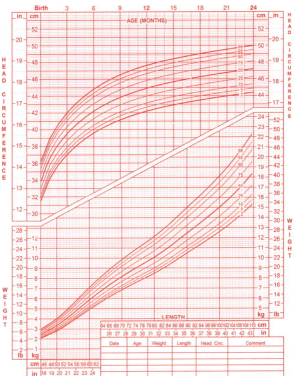

Birth to 24 months: Girls
Head circumference-for-age and
Weight-for-length percentiles

NAME _____

RECORD # _____

Published by the Centers for Disease Control and Prevention, November 1, 2009
SOURCE: WHO Child Growth Standards (http://www.who.int/childgrowth/en)

PEDS
ASSESS

CDC Growth Charts

Use these charts for children from 2 to 20 years of age.

Published May 30, 2000 (modified 11/21/00). Source: Developed by the National Center for Health Statistics in collaboration with the National Center for Chronic Disease Prevention and Health Promotion (2000). http://www.cdc.gov/growthcharts. Retrieved from http://www.cdc.gov/growthcharts/clinical_charts.htm.

BMI Calculation and Interpretation

According to CDC: BMI is used as a screening tool to identify possible weight problems for children. CDC and the American Academy of Pediatrics (AAP) recommend the use of BMI to screen for overweight and obesity in children beginning at 2 years old.

For children, BMI is used to screen for obesity, overweight, healthy weight, or underweight. However, BMI is not a diagnostic tool. For example, a child may have a high BMI for age and gender, but to determine whether excess fat is a problem, a health-care provider would need to perform further assessments. These assessments might include skinfold thickness measurements, evaluations of diet, physical activity, family history, and other appropriate health screenings.

First, BMI is calculated according to instructions below, then, BMI must be compared with age- and gender-specific data on the following percentile based charts.

First, calculate BMI using one of the following formulas:

Measurement Units	Formula and Calculation
Kilograms and meters (or centimeters)	Formula: weight (kg)/[height (m)]^2 With the metric system, the formula for BMI is weight in kilograms divided by height in meters squared. Because height is commonly measured in centimeters, an alternate calculation formula, dividing the weight in kilograms by the height in centimeters squared, and then multiplying the result by 10,000, can be used.
Pounds and inches	Formula: weight (lb)/[height (in)]$^2 \times 703$ When using English measurements, ounces (oz) and fractions must be changed to decimal values. Then, calculate BMI by dividing weight in pounds (lb) by height in inches (in) squared and multiplying by a conversion factor of 703.

Next, to determine BMI percentile, plot the child's BMI on the appropriate percentile chart (see following BMI percentile charts).
- Alternative method for calculating BMI and BMI-for-age percentile: use BMI calculator at the following Web site: http://nccd.cdc.gov/dnpabmi/Calculator.aspx

Published May 30, 2000 (modified 10/16/00). Source: Developed by the National Center for Health Statistics in collaboration with the National Center for Chronic Disease Prevention and Health Promotion (2000). http://www.cdc.gov/growthcharts. Retrieved from http://www.cdc.gov/growthcharts/clinical_charts.htm.

PEDS
ASSESS

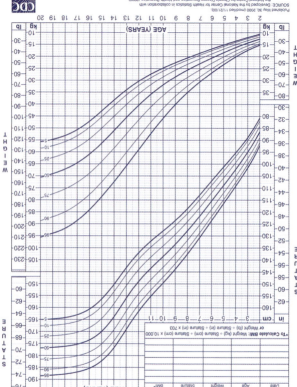

Stature-for-age and Weight-for-age percentiles

2 to 20 years: Boys

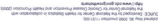

205

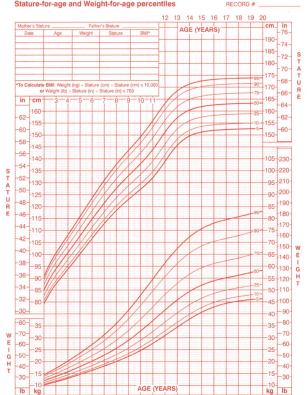

2 to 20 years: Girls
Stature-for-age and Weight-for-age percentiles

NAME _____

RECORD # _____

Mother's Stature _____ Father's Stature _____

Date	Age	Weight	Stature	BMI*

*To Calculate BMI: Weight (kg) ÷ Stature (cm) ÷ Stature (cm) x 10,000
or Weight (lb) ÷ Stature (in) ÷ Stature (in) x 703

AGE (YEARS)

STATURE

WEIGHT

Published May 30, 2000 (modified 11/21/00).
SOURCE: Developed by the National Center for Health Statistics in collaboration with
the National Center for Chronic Disease Prevention and Health Promotion (2000).
http://www.cdc.gov/growthcharts

CDC
SAFER • HEALTHIER • PEOPLE™

PEDS
ASSESS

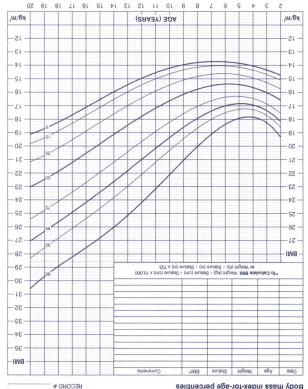

Body mass index-for-age percentiles

NAME

RECORD #

2 to 20 years: Boys

*To Calculate BMI: Weight (kg) ÷ Stature (cm) ÷ Stature (cm) x 10,000
or Weight (lb) ÷ Stature (in) ÷ Stature (in) x 703

Date	Age	Weight	Stature	BMI*	Comments

BMI

AGE (YEARS)

kg/m²

Published May 30, 2000 (modified 10/16/00).

SOURCE: Developed by the National Center for Health Statistics in collaboration with
the National Center for Chronic Disease Prevention and Health Promotion (2000).
http://www.cdc.gov/growthcharts

2 to 20 years: Girls
Body mass index-for-age percentiles

NAME _____

RECORD # _____

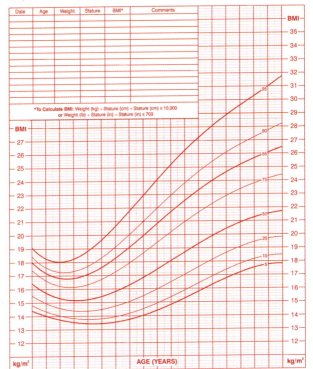

Date	Age	Weight	Stature	BMI*	Comments

*To Calculate BMI: Weight (kg) ÷ Stature (cm) ÷ Stature (cm) x 10,000
or Weight (lb) ÷ Stature (in) ÷ Stature (in) x 703

AGE (YEARS)

BMI — kg/m²

Published May 30, 2000 (modified 10/16/00).
SOURCE: Developed by the National Center for Health Statistics in collaboration with
the National Center for Chronic Disease Prevention and Health Promotion (2000).
http://www.cdc.gov/growthcharts

CDC
SAFER • HEALTHIER • PEOPLE™

PEDS ASSESS

Calculate BMI-for-age weight status categories and corresponding percentiles:

Weight Status Category	Percentile Range
Underweight	Less than the 5th percentile
Healthy weight	5th percentile to less than the 85th percentile
Overweight	85th percentile to less than the 95th percentile for children and teens of same age and gender
Obese	Equal to or greater than the 95th percentile for children and teens of same age and gender

Data from http://www.cdc.gov/healthyweight/assessing/bmi/childrens_bmi/about_childrens_bmi.html.

Dentition

The Primary Teeth

Upper Teeth	Erupt
Central Incisor	8–12 Months
Lateral Incisor	9–13 Months
Canine (Cuspid)	16–22 Months
First Molar	13–19 Months
Second Molar	25–33 Months

Child

Lower Teeth

Second Molar	23–31 Months
First Molar	14–18 Months
Canine (Cuspid)	17–23 Months
Lateral Incisor	10–16 Months
Central Incisor	6–10 Months

Adult

Upper Jaw

Lower Jaw

The Permanent Teeth

1. Central incisor
2. Lateral Incisor
3. Canine
4. 1st Premolar
5. 2nd Premolar
6. 1st Molar
7. 2nd Molar
8. 3rd Molar (wisdom teeth)

Assessment of Acutely Ill or Hospitalized Child

Assessment Type	Findings
First assess ABCs (airway, breathing, circulation) and then perform relevant portions of the assessment based on the child's condition and known or suspected diagnosis	Expected findings in black font; pathological findings and possible indications in red font
Airway/Oxygenation*	
*Also see "O_2 saturation" under Circulation	
Observe patency of airway	• Airway patent and free of foreign body and excess mucus • Airway impaired by foreign body, mucus, inflammation, or bronchospasm; note that smoke inhalation may cause inflammation • Gurgling or adventitious breath sounds may indicate partial obstruction of airway
Listen	• Respirations quiet • Audible **wheezes** may indicate bronchospasm, bronchiolitis, or foreign body in airway; wheezes should be recorded as inspiratory or expiratory or biphasic (both) • **Expiratory grunt** indicates an effort to increase end-expiratory pressure in order to keep alveoli expanded and to increase alveolar gas exchange • No pursed-lip breathing • Older children may purse lips during expiration in an attempt to keep the airway open for a longer period

Continued

Assessment of Acutely Ill or Hospitalized Child—cont'd

Assessment Type	Findings

	• No stridor
	  • **Acute inspiratory stridor** (a grating or crowing sound) is a sign of upper airway obstruction; above the glottis—usually croup
	  • **Chronic inspiratory stridor** is a sign of laryngomalacia—a congenital abnormality in which the laryngeal soft tissue collapses
	  • **Expiratory stridor** is a sign of obstruction in the lower trachea
	  • **Biphasic stridor** may indicate swelling in the cricoid cartilage that surrounds the trachea
	  • Drooling may indicate airway obstruction
	  • Restlessness is an EARLY sign of air hunger

Smell Assess trauma or burn victims for smoky odor to breath	• No smoky odor to breath • Smoky odor to breath may indicate smoke inhalation and indicates the need to observe for delayed airway swelling
Breathing	
Observe rate, rhythm, and effort	• Respiratory rate even with rate appropriate for age (see respiratory rate table on p 185) • Irregular respiratory rate or apnea may indicate airway obstruction, pain, or neurological abnormality • Note that periodic breathing (no breathing for 15–20 seconds) is common in young infants and is not known to be associated with pathology

Continued

PEDS ACUTE

Continued

Assessment of Acutely Ill or Hospitalized Child—cont'd

Assessment Type	Findings

	• No soft tissue retractions or flaring of nostrils
	• Soft tissue retractions, head bobbing, or flaring of the nostrils indicate increased work of breathing; retractions may be one or more of the following types:
	  • Intercostal (between ribs)
	  • Subcostal (under ribs)
	  • Suprasternal (above sternum)
	  • Substernal (under sternum)
	  • Supraclavicular (above clavicle)
	• Shallow respirations may indicate fatigue and need for assisted ventilation; this may occur in infant with RSV infection

Auscultate lungs, all lobes; anterior and posterior
 	
Right middle lobe is auscultated in the right axilla
	• **Bronchial sounds** are loud and high-pitched hollow sounds that are heard over the upper anterior chest
	• **Bronchovesicular sounds** are softer tubular sounds heard in the anterior central chest and between the scapula in the posterior chest
	• **Vesicular sounds** are soft blowing sounds heard throughout peripheral lung fields
	• **Adventitious sounds (abnormal)** heard with auscultation may indicate foreign body or mucus in airway, bronchiolitis, asthma, pneumonia, or other pathology; child may have more than one type of adventitious sound such as the following:
	  • **Rales:** Crackling sound; common in pneumonia
	  • **Rhonchi:** Coarse sounds; often clear with coughing
	  • **Wheezing, musical, or sibilant rales:** Whistling sounds; common with asthma and bronchiolitis

Assessment of Acutely Ill or Hospitalized Child—cont'd

Assessment Type	Findings
	Note that when mucus has collected in the pharynx or upper airway, a loud rhonchi-like sound may be transmitted and heard throughout the lung fields during auscultation; place the stethoscope on the child's neck to determine whether this has happened; finding an indication of mucus in the upper airway does not eliminate the possibility of lung pathology; it is possible for a child to have both excess mucus in the upper airway AND lung pathology; adventitious sounds caused only by mucus in the upper airway will clear when the child coughs

Observe activity and feeding	• Child active, playing, or interacting appropriately with environment and eating well
	  • In infants, decreased oxygenation may result in hunger and irritability due to short periods of frequent feeding that are interrupted by the need to rest
	  • Older child may lean forward in "tripod position" during shortness of breath; this position lessens pressure on diaphragm and maximizes chest expansion

Circulation	

Auscultate apical pulse for rate, rhythm, and abnormal sounds	• Apical pulse has regular rhythm, and rate is appropriate for age (see Vital Signs chart on p 166)
	  • Note that child's heart rate and rhythm will vary with respiratory effort
	• No murmur heard
	  • A murmur is a blowing sound that is heard between "lub" and "dup" (systolic murmur) or between "dup" and "lub" (diastolic murmur); murmurs indicate turbulent blood flow or movement of blood under increased pressure; see p 180 for grading of murmurs

Continued

PEDS
ACUTE

Assessment of Acutely Ill or Hospitalized Child—cont'd

Assessment Type	Findings
Palpate peripheral pulses and perfusion	• Pulses equal in all extremities (see illustration on p 195 for location of pulses) • Capillary refill is brisk in fingers and toes
Observe O_2 saturation (pulse oximetry) if indicated	• O_2 saturation = 95% or above • O_2 saturation of less than 95% indicates decreased oxygenation of tissue • Note: A pulse oximeter indicates the amount of hemoglobin that is saturated with oxygen; thus, an anemic child may have a "false high" O_2 saturation because it takes less oxygen to saturate less hemoglobin
Measure blood pressure (BP)	• Blood pressure appropriate for gender and age (see table on pp 187–194) • Note: Elasticity of a child's blood vessels means that decreased blood pressure may not occur in early shock
Temperature	

Measure using age appropriate method and device	• Temperature appropriate for assessment site:
	  • Oral temperature is near 98.6°F or 37°C in most children
	  • Ear or rectal temperature is near 99.6°F; axillary temperature is near 97.6°F
	  • Note that small, premature infants normally have little variation in temp based on assessment site
	• Elevated temperature may indicate infection
	• In a newborn or young infant, a subnormal body *or* an elevated temperature and poor feeding are important indicators of sepsis

Lymph Nodes	
Palpate with fingertips, using a circular motion	• Lymph nodes are nonpalpable (see figure on p 196 for location of lymph nodes) • Lymph nodes that are enlarged, tender, and mobile are signs of infection

Continued

Assessment of Acutely Ill or Hospitalized Child—cont'd

Assessment Type	Findings
	• Lymph nodes that are nontender and nonmobile may be attached to an underlying tumor • Small, 1- to 2-mm size nodes that are nontender are common in young children; referred to as "shotty" nodes and thought to be indicators of past infection

Neurological Status

Assessment Type	Findings
Observe behavior and test reflexes	• Behavior and reflex responses appropriate for stimuli
Test using Glasgow Coma Scale if child has a neurological injury	• Glasgow Coma Score (see p 224)
Perform tests for meningeal irritation (meningitis is an example) if child is febrile and diagnosis has not been established	
• Flex neck to move the head forward	• Neck moves without pain, stiffness, or flexion of the legs • Stiffness of neck movement may indicate meningeal irritation (meningitis) • Flexion of hip and knee during neck flexion is an indicator of meningeal irritation and is termed a positive Brudzinski sign
• Flex the hip and knee, then, attempt passive extension of the knee	• Knee extends to approximately 180° without pain • Pain with extension of knee to 180° is an indicator of meningeal irritation and is termed a positive Kernig sign

Continued

PEDS ACUTE

Assessment of Acutely Ill or Hospitalized Child—cont'd

Assessment Type	Findings
Mouth and Pharynx	

Observe	• Mucous membranes pink without lesions
	  • White coating that cannot be removed from tongue or mucous membranes may indicate thrush, a candidal infection that is common in children who are immunosuppressed or who are taking antibiotics
	  • Mucosal ulcers may indicate immunosuppression, autoimmune disease, or viral infection
	• Pharynx pink without exudate or swelling of pharynx or tonsils
	  • Pharyngeal or tonsillar redness, exudate, or enlargement may indicate viral or bacterial infection

Skin	

Observe for skin temperature and hydration
If abdomen is distended, check skin turgor in another body area such as over sternum or over tibia
	• Skin warm and slightly moist
	• Skin has elastic turgor
	  • Skin recoils slowly or "tents" when lightly pinched, indicating dehydration
	    • Note: Because of a large body surface area, young children rapidly become dehydrated
	  • Taut, shining skin indicates swelling or edema that my be caused by excess IV fluid, kidney malfunction, or heart failure

Observe skin for irritation, breakdown, lesions, and pressure areas; include diaper area inspection in children who are not toilet-trained	• Skin is intact and free of lesions, including diaper area
	  • If reddened areas or skin breakdown is observed, note and record size, characteristics, and number of lesions as well as distribution (see Skin Lesion table on p 169)
	  • Notes:
	    • Ill children are prone to have diaper dermatitis—always assess for this

Continued

Assessment of Acutely Ill or Hospitalized Child—cont'd

Assessment Type	Findings
	• Children who have been taking antibiotics have an increased risk for a candidal diaper rash; this rash often appears beefy red with satellite lesions
	• Irritation or pressure areas may form when a child is on bed rest, in one position, for extended periods of time, or when tape or equipment is in constant contact with skin; children with edema or swelling and those who are being treated with topical steroids are at higher risk for skin breakdown
	• Pustules with honey-colored crust are characteristic of impetigo, a common skin infection that is highly contagious
	• A sandpaper-like rash on the trunk is characteristic of scarlet fever or scarlatina; caused by strep pharyngitis
	• Desquamation (peeling) of skin on palms of hands, feet, and diaper area may occur after Kawasaki disease or strep infection
	• Circular lesions with central clearing are characteristic of tinea, or ringworm, which is caused by a fungus
	• Roseola is a common viral condition that occurs in children ages 6 mo to 3 yr; the child has high fever and possibly a mild upper respiratory illness (URI) and cervical lymphadenopathy for several days, followed by lower or normal temperature and a macular or papular pinkish-red rash that begins on the trunk and may spread over the entire body; the rash blanches when pressure is applied, and individual spots may appear to be surrounded by halos

Continued

Assessment of Acutely Ill or Hospitalized Child—cont'd

Assessment Type	Findings
Abdomen	
Observe	• Abdomen flat without visible peristalsis • Abdominal distention may indicate obstruction, heart failure, internal bleeding, or gastrointestinal infection • Visible peristalsis may indicate obstruction • An olive-shaped mass in the upper abdomen, accompanied by vomiting, may indicate pyloric stenosis
Auscultate	• Bowel sounds heard in four quadrants • Hyperactive or absent bowel sounds may indicate infection or obstruction
Palpate abdomen for masses	• No palpable masses • Palpable mass; record location and approximate palpable size
Palpate liver	• Edge of liver may be palpable below right costal margin (RCM) • Liver more than 2 cm below RCM may indicate heart failure, hepatitis, biliary atresia, and other illnesses
Palpate spleen	• Spleen usually not palpable • Spleen that is palpable in left upper quadrant may occur in a child with infectious mononucleosis (as part of the lymphatic system) or in a child with sickle cell anemia (as an organ that removes defective red blood cells)
Perform scratch test • Used to estimate size of the liver or spleen, the scratch test is a useful alternative to abdominal percussion	• A dull sound is heard over the organ and a hollow sound beyond the edges of the organ; see previous palpation entries for comments on organ size • Note that a full bowel may distort test sounds

Continued

Assessment of Acutely Ill or Hospitalized Child—cont'd

Assessment Type	Findings
• Use one hand to place stethoscope over the organ (liver or spleen) while using the index finger of the opposite hand to make light scratching movements over the organ; move stethoscope toward each edge of the organ while continuing scratching motion near the stethoscope	

Extremities

Palpate each extremity for warmth and mobility while assessing for pain	• All extremities pink, warm, and mobile without painful movement • Limited movement may occur with cerebral palsy or with the formation of contractures following trauma • Pain in joints may indicate Lyme disease, rheumatoid arthritis, infection, or rheumatic fever, which is an autoimmune reaction to a strep infection

Continued

PEDS
ACUTE

Assessment of Acutely Ill or Hospitalized Child—cont'd

Assessment Type	Findings
Observe, following treatments and procedures, to be certain that no tourniquets or inappropriate restraints have been left on any extremity and no needles or syringes have been left in the bed	No tourniquets, nonessential restraints, or other nonessential medical devices left in the child's bed Note: When more than one attempt has been made to start an IV, a forgotten tourniquet may be inadvertently left on an extremity or small medical devices (such as needles or caps) may be hidden under sheets or other bedding
Observe and palpate extremities for evidence of fracture after suspected or validated traumatic injury	• No report of pain when extremities are palpated • No swelling, false motion (movement at a point where there is normally no motion), or obvious deformity of extremities • No crepitation (grating or popping sound) • Peripheral pulses strong • Pain, deformity, swelling, false motion, or crepitation may occur with fracture (see p •• for illustration of fracture types)
Elimination	
Observe and record time, size, color, and consistency of stools and recent frequency of bowel elimination	• Stools brown and soft • Red blood-tinged stools indicate bleeding from lower gastrointestinal (GI) tract or rectal area • Note: Cranberry-colored stools should be guaiac-tested for blood; consumption of red gelatin may cause cranberry-colored stools in child with diarrhea • Black stools may indicate GI bleeding (from upper GI tract) or may be caused by supplemental iron intake • Pale stools may indicate liver pathology • Fatty stools (steatorrhea) may indicate high-fat diet, celiac disease, or cystic fibrosis

Continued

Assessment of Acutely Ill or Hospitalized Child—cont'd

Assessment Type	Findings
Observe color and frequency of urination	• Urine pale yellow with at least four urine voidings per day • Dark urine in a child most often indicates dehydration
Measure urine specific gravity (s.g.) if indicated (especially if child has had vomiting or diarrhea or has been without fluid intake for longer than usual)	• Urine s.g. of 1.002–1.028 • Urine s.g. that is higher than 1.023 and that does not decrease in response to conservative treatment (oral fluids) may indicate need for intravenous fluids • High urine s.g. may indicate contamination or high urine glucose content

Secretions/Drainage

Observe and record amount, color, and consistency of nasal mucus secretions and sputum	• Mucus is scant and clear • Profuse amounts of clear mucus secretions may indicate irritation and/or allergy • Bloody mucus or sputum may indicate trauma, infection, or a bleeding disorder • Green or yellow mucus may indicate infection • Note that respiratory tract mucus may be slightly yellow during a viral infection but that prolonged yellow or green secretions generally indicate a bacterial infection; viral infections may predispose to bacterial infections
Observe drainage from wounds or lesions	• Wound or lesion drainage is serous (pale yellow and thin) or serosanguineous (a mixture of serous and bloody secretions) • Dark yellow or greenish wound or lesion drainage may indicate bacterial infection

Continued

PEDS ACUTE

Assessment of Acutely Ill or Hospitalized Child—cont'd

Assessment Type	Findings
Appetite and Activity	
Observe intake	• Child eating, sleeping, playing, and showing interest in surroundings • Failure to eat, sleep, play, or show an interest indicates illness and may precede changes in vital signs
Environment, Equipment, and Medical Devices	
Observe environment for safety hazards, including possible need for bubble-top crib	• Side rails up without indication that child may climb out of crib • Infants and toddlers who are able to pull to a standing position may be able to climb over crib rails and should be placed in a bubble top bed if they will be left unattended
Observe bedding and immediate area for bottles, cups, medications, tubing, tourniquets, needles, needle caps, writing pens, paper, etc., that may have been accidently left in child's bed	• No unsafe objects in child's bed or within reach • No excess linens in bed
Observe appearance, function, and readings of medical devices in room	• Monitors indicate that vital signs are appropriate for age • Feeding tube properly placed • GI contents can be aspirated from nasogastric (NG) tube, or small quantity of air forced into tube can be heard or palpated over gastric area • Note: Before each feeding, check back of infant's mouth where NG tube can be regurgitated and displaced

Continued

Assessment of Acutely Ill or Hospitalized Child—cont'd

Assessment Type	Findings
	• IV delivering prescribed fluids at prescribed rate • No swelling or redness at IV site • Foley catheter draining clear pale yellow urine • Oxygen and respiratory devices operating at prescribed settings • Suction equipment operational and clean

Specialized Assessment Tools

The following four assessment tools are for use in children with traumatic injury.

Pediatric Trauma Score

Assessment	Score +2	Score +1	Score −1
Weight	>20 kg	10–20 kg	<10 kg
Airway	Normal	Maintainable	Invasive (intubated)
Systolic blood pressure	>90 mm Hg	50–90 mm Hg	<50 mm Hg
Mental status	Awake	Obtunded	Comatose
Open wound	None	Minor	Major
Skeletal trauma	None	Closed fracture	Open or multiple fractures

Pediatric Trauma Score <8 = significant mortality risk.
Data from Ford E.G., Andrassy R.J. (1994). *Pediatric Trauma Initial Assessment and Management.* Philadelphia: W.B. Saunders, p. 112.

Glasgow Coma Scale for Infants and Toddlers

Description	Score
Eye Opening	
Spontaneous	4
To sounds and speech	3
To pain	2
None	1
Verbal Response—Infant	
Smiles, interacts, follows objects	5
Cries, consolable	4
Cries, inconsistently consolable	3
Cries, inconsolable	2
No response	1
Verbal Response—Toddler	
Interacts appropriately	5
Interacts but confused	4
Moans, uses inappropriate words	3
Incomprehensible sounds	2
No response	1
Best Motor Response	
Obeys command to move body part	6
Localized pain	5
Tries to remove painful stimuli	4
Flexes arm in response to pain	3
Extends arm in response to pain	2
No response	1

Types of Fractures

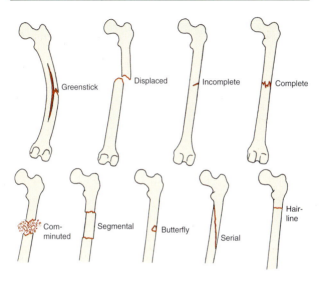

Greenstick

Displaced

Incomplete

Complete

Com-minuted

Segmental

Butterfly

Serial

Hair-line

Estimation of Burned Body Surface Area in Children

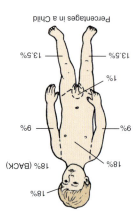

Percentages in a Child

13.5%   13.5%

1%

9%   9%

18% (BACK)   18%

18%

Conditions That Commonly Require Pediatric Hospital Admission

Asthma

Pathophysiology
Airway stimuli result in spasms and edema of the bronchi and bronchioles with increased production and viscosity of mucus. Air is trapped distal to the resulting obstruction. Alveolar gas exchange is impaired. There is a familial predisposition to asthma.

Possible Causes of Acute Exacerbation
- Respiratory infection
- Allergens
- Respiratory irritants such as smoke, dust, or cold air
- Exercise
- Emotional stress

Signs and Symptoms
- Wheezing
- Dyspnea
- Uncontrollable cough
- Nasal flaring
- Musical rales
- Anxiety

Medical Treatment
- Bronchodilators (such as Albuterol)
- Epinephrine
- Corticosteroids
- Expectorants
- Antibiotics if infection is present

Nursing Diagnoses
- Ineffective airway clearance
- Impaired gas exchange
- Activity intolerance
- Anxiety

Nursing Implications
- Wash hands before and after care
- Monitor vital signs and report marked changes

- Monitor oxygen saturation (O_2 sat)
- Monitor oral intake
- Monitor hydration
- Encourage oral fluid intake
- Administer ordered medications and monitor for side effects
- Monitor IV fluids type and rate
- Administer prescribed medications and monitor for side effects and adverse reactions
- Auscultate respiratory sounds, listening for failure to move air and for adventitious sounds
  - Report change in intensity or duration of breath sounds
- Plan care to allow for uninterrupted periods of rest
- Educate regarding avoidance of exacerbations

Prognosis
About half of children will outgrow exacerbations. Persistent asthma may lead to development of chronic obstructive pulmonary disease (COPD).

Bronchiolitis

Pathophysiology
Swelling of the small airways leads to hyperinflations distal to the obstructions. Resultant pneumonitis and patchy areas of atelectasis may be present. Most common in children younger than 2 years. Prematurity increases the risk for condition.

Possible Causes
- Respiratory infection
  - RSV infection in most cases
  - Adenovirus
  - Parainfluenza virus

Signs and Symptoms
- Barrel-shaped chest
- Retractions
- Nasal flaring
- Tachypnea
- Cough
- Wheezing (mimics asthma)
- Anorexia
- Fever

Medical Treatment

- Bronchodilators
- Corticosteroids
- High humidity air (croup tent)
- Supplemental oxygen to maintain $Sao_2 \geq 95\%$
- Increased fluid intake at 1½ times maintenance (see Pediatric Fluid Calculation on p 259)

Nursing Diagnoses

- Ineffective breathing pattern
- Ineffective airway clearance
- Impaired gas exchange
- Potential fluid volume deficit
- Anxiety

Nursing Implications

- Hand washing is the most effective prevention against RSV and its spread
- Suction as needed
- Monitor and maintain hydration
- Monitor oxygen saturation
- Provide supplemental oxygen if indicated
- Pregnant women should be warned that RSV may be teratogenic
- Educate all visitors regarding hand washing

Prognosis

Normal lung function is usually recovered after several weeks. Lung problems may persist for years. There is an increased incidence of asthma.

Croup (Laryngotracheobronchitis)

Pathophysiology

Inflammation and spasm of the larynx, trachea, and bronchi.

Cause

Viral infection, usually parainfluenza, but may also be caused by RSV, influenza, or bacterial infection.

Signs and Symptoms

Seal-like barking cough and inspiratory stridor, x-ray may show narrowing of the trachea (subglottic) or the "steeple sign."

Medical Treatment
- Hydration
- Humidified air
- Corticosteroids
- Oxygen
- Racemic epinephrine

Nursing Diagnoses
- Ineffective airway clearance
- Fluid volume deficit
- Fear

Nursing Implications
- Wash hands before and after care
- Close monitoring of vital signs
- Monitor respiratory effort
- Monitor oxygen saturation (pulse oximeter)
- Keep environment calm
- Ensure adequate fluid intake
- Explain all procedures to family
- If possible, allow a parent or caregiver to room in with child

Prognosis
- Good with prompt treatment

Cystic Fibrosis

Pathophysiology
Inherited autosomal recessive disease of the lungs, pancreas, urogenital system, skeleton, and skin. Mucus secretions are thick, leading to respiratory infections, poor food absorption, and constipation. Excess salt is lost via sweat. There is progressive lung dysfunction.

Common Causes of Acute Illness
- Respiratory infection
- GI malfunction such as constipation

Signs and Symptoms
- Nasal polyps
- Failure to thrive
- Voracious appetite
- Dyspnea, cough

- Excess salt in sweat
- Thick mucus secretions
- Frequent respiratory infections
- Bulky, foul-smelling stools
- Constipation
- Meconium ileus (failure to pass meconium) in newborns
- Rectal prolapse

Medical Treatment
- Annual influenza immunization
- Pneumococcal vaccination
- Oral pancreatic enzymes
- Antibiotics during infections
- Humidified air
- Chest physiotherapy (percussion and postural drainage)

Nursing Diagnoses
- Ineffective airway clearance
- Potential for infection
- Altered nutrition, less than body requirements
- Risk for electrolyte imbalance
- Risk for constipation
- Knowledge deficit
- Fear
- Diversional activity deficit
- Sleep pattern disturbance

Nursing Implications
- Wash hands before and after care
- Administer medications and monitor for side effects
  - Note: Frequent and prolonged use of antibiotics may decrease intestinal bacterial synthesis of vitamin K and impair blood clotting
- IV fluids as ordered
- Ensure compatibility of IV antibiotics
- Encourage oral fluid intake
- Plan care, including chest physiotherapy, to allow for uninterrupted periods of rest
- Plan chest physiotherapy so that it does not occur near meal times (cough and mucus expectoration may decrease appetite)
- Offer extra snacks with salt to taste; as a result of poor food absorption, extra calories are needed
- Referral to support groups

Prognosis
Average life span is 35 years. Males generally survive longer than females.

Dehydration

Pathology
Children have less body fluid reserve than adults and have a larger body surface area that allows more fluid to be lost through perspiration. The GI tract is proportionately longer in children, leading to relatively greater fluid loss. Immature kidneys mean that a child is less able to conserve electrolytes. In early dehydration, fluid loss is both intracellular and extracellular. In chronic dehydration, fluid loss is predominantly cellular. Fluid loss may result in shock, acidosis, or alkalosis, kidney and brain damage, and death.

Common Causes of Dehydration
■ Viral or bacterial infection that results in vomiting and/or diarrhea
■ Extensive burns
■ Diabetic ketoacidosis

Severity of Dehydration	Signs
	(Child should be assessed for signs and findings recorded at least every 8 hours, when assessing child who is hospitalized for treatment of dehydration)
Mild	Wt loss 3%–5% of body weight Vital signs normal Mucous membranes normal Tears present Fontanel normal Behavior normal Urine output decreased
Moderate	Wt loss 6%–10% of body weight BP may be decreased Mucous membranes dry Tears decreased Fontanel may be sunken Irritable Urine output markedly decreased

Continued

Severity of Dehydration	Signs
Severe	Wt loss 10%–15% of body weight BP may be markedly decreased Mucous membranes very dry No tears Fontanel sunken Very irritable or lethargic Urine output scant or absent

Signs and Symptoms
May include the following:
- Poor skin turgor
- Lack of tears
- Sunken anterior fontanel
- Weight loss\decreased urine output
- Increased urine specific gravity (greater than 1.023)

Medical Treatment
May include the following:
- Oral rehydration solutions (ORS)
- IV fluids and electrolytes if fluids cannot be ingested or retained
- IV fluid formula:
  - First 8 hours = maintenance fluids + half the estimated fluid deficit Use 1 kg of weight loss to represent 1000 mL of fluid loss (see Pediatric Maintenance Fluid Calculation on p 259)
  - Next 24–48 hours = maintenance fluids + remaining estimated fluid deficit is added to maintenance fluid

Nursing Care
May include the following:
- Wash hands before and after care
- Weigh on admission to estimate severity of dehydration (see table on p 232)
- Continue to assess hydration status, e.g., turgor, mucous membranes
- Wear gloves when changing diapers
- Adhere to ordered feeding type and times
- If oral feedings induce vomiting most of ingested fluids, or if volume of stools is increased with feeding, notify physician so that IV fluids may be initiated or appropriate rate of IV flow may be determined

PEDS
ACUTE

- Monitor IV fluids type and control appropriate rate of flow
  - Note: Potassium (K⁺) is not added to IV fluids until after the child voids (voiding indicates presence of kidney function)
- Assess and record size, color, and consistency of all vomitus and stools
- Weigh diapers using gram scale (subtract weight of dry diaper)
  - 1 gram in wt equals 1 mL of urine or liquid stool
  - Goal is to achieve 0.5 to 1 mL/h urinary output for each kilogram of body wt
- Keep diaper area clean and inspect for skin breakdown with each diaper change
- Be aware that in children blood vessels adapt quickly to intravascular fluid loss, so decreased blood pressure is not a reliable indication of early shock in young children
- Communicate to family and other caregivers that the nurse needs to be made aware of all elimination
- Educate all visitors regarding hand washing
- Notify physician of acute change in condition

Prognosis
Good with rehydration.

Diabetes Mellitus (DM)

Pathophysiology
A group of syndromes characterized by the inability to metabolize carbohydrates.

- Type 1 DM is caused by autoimmune destruction of the insulin-secreting cells of the pancreas and results in failure of the pancreas to produce insulin
- Type 2 DM may result from insufficient insulin production and/or body cellular resistance to the effects of insulin; excess body weight increases the risk for type 2 DM
- Diagnosis requires at least one of the following:
  - Fasting plasma glucose level exceeds 126 mg/dL on two occasions
  - Random glucose levels exceed 200 mg/dL
  - 2-hour oral glucose tolerance test is 200 mg/dL or higher

Signs and Symptoms
May include the following:
- Hyperglycemia
- Polydipsia (excessive thirst)

- Polyuria (excessive urination)
- Polyphagia (excessive hunger)
- Anorexia (loss of appetite)
- Weight loss (type 1)
- Ketones in urine

Medical Treatment

May include the following:

- Medications that replace insulin, stimulate insulin secretion, or decrease insulin resistance
- Monitor for complications
- Monitor blood glucose and A1C
- In patients with type 1 diabetes, regular laboratory testing for other autoimmune conditions, e.g., Graves' disease and celiac disease
- Regular dilated eye examinations
- ACE inhibitor for blood pressure and to preserve renal function

Nursing Diagnoses

May include the following:

- Altered nutrition, less than or more than body requirements
- Unstable blood glucose
- Alteration in elimination
- Potential fluid volume deficit
- Fatigue
- Risk for infection
- Knowledge deficit
- Multiple psychosocial diagnoses

Nursing Implications

- Wash hands before and after care
- Monitor blood glucose
- Monitor for the following:
  - **Signs of Hypoglycemia**—low blood sugar
    - Hunger
    - Shakiness
    - Sweating
    - Headache
    - Pallor
    - Tingling around mouth
  - **Signs of Hyperglycemia**—high blood sugar
    - Blurring of vision
    - Drowsiness

- Frequent urination
- Polydipsia
- **Signs of Ketoacidosis**—(most common in patients with type 1 diabetes) when the body does not have enough insulin to use glucose or if insufficient glucose is consumed for energy, it may respond by burning fat for energy; fat breakdown results in ketones, which are acids, building up in the blood and appearing in the urine; ketoacidosis can result in diabetic coma and death
  - High level of urine ketones
  - High level of blood glucose and urine ketones
  - Vomiting when urine ketones are high
  - Abdominal pain
  - Fatigue
  - Dry or flushed skin
  - Respirations that are short and shallow, followed by respirations that are deep and labored (Kussmaul respirations) as body attempts to "blow off" CO_2
  - Fruity odor on breath
  - Confusion
- **Signs of Hyperosmolar Nonketotic Coma**—(most common in type 2 diabetes) occurs most often when the patient is stressed or ill with an infection or after a myocardial infarction or other illness; insulin deficiency leads to elevated blood glucose that may result in diabetic coma without ketosis (fat breakdown); this is different from diabetic ketoacidosis in which there is no insulin
  - Polydipsia (excess thirst)
  - Polyuria (excess urination)
  - Dehydration
  - Shock
- Thoroughly assess feet, including soles and between toes
- Assess hydration
- Teach patient and family regarding diet, monitoring of blood glucose, signs and symptoms and management of hypoglycemia, importance of regular exercise, signs and symptoms of infection, foot care, compliance with medical regimen, medication side effects, importance of eye examinations, home blood pressure monitoring, and when to contact the health-care provider
- Teach signs of hypoglycemia and hyperglycemia and treatment of each
- Provide encouragement and emotional support for patient and family

Prognosis

Varies with type of diabetes, age of onset, compliance, and complicating factors. Poor glucose and blood pressure control increase the risk for complications and early mortality. Excess body weight increases the risk for complications in patients with type 2 diabetes.

Meningitis

Pathophysiology

Inflammation of the meninges (covering) of the spinal cord and/or brain, usually caused by an infection, either viral or bacterial.

Usual Causes

- Infection
  - Viral
  - Bacterial (bacterial meningitis is a medical emergency that may result in death if not quickly treated with antibiotics)

Signs and Symptoms

May include the following:
- Fever
- Vomiting
- Headache
- Nuchal (neck) rigidity to flexion
- Positive Kernig sign (see p 215)
- Positive Brudzinski sign (see p 215)
- Irritability
- Photosensitivity
- Seizures

Medical Treatment

May include the following:
- IV antibiotics
- IV dexamethasone
- Antipyretics

Nursing Diagnoses

May include the following:
- Pain
- Sensory perception alteration
- Risk for ineffective cerebral tissue perfusion
- Hyperthermia

PEDS ACUTE

■ Risk for trauma/suffocation (related to alternations in consciousness and risk for seizures)

Nursing Implications

May include the following:

■ Frequent vital sign and neuro checks
■ Administer medications as ordered, including prn medications for fever and discomfort
■ Monitor for side effects and adverse reactions to medications
■ Assess compatibility of IV medications
■ Monitor I&O—watch for signs of inappropriate secretion of antidiuretic hormone (ISADH) caused by excess release of diuretic hormone (vasopressin) from the posterior pituitary, which may result in hyponatremia and fluid overload
■ Prevention of bacterial meningitis by encouraging routine immunization for *Haemophilus influenzae* (Hib) and pneumococcus (Prevnar) (use of this immunization has also resulted in a decrease in the incidence of epiglottitis)

Prognosis

Varies depending on type and age of child; brain damage and hearing impairment may occur; bacterial meningitis has a mortality rate of 10% to 40%.

Pneumonia

Pathophysiology

Infection and inflammation of the lungs lead to alveolar edema that promotes spread of the infecting organism. Solidification of the infected lobe(s) is caused by exudates (referred to as *consolidation* in radiology reports).

Usual Causes

■ Aspiration
■ Fluid stasis
■ Infection
  ■ Bacterial
  ■ Viral

Signs and Symptoms

May include the following:

■ Fever
■ Chills

- Cough
- Dyspnea
- Tachypnea
- Tachycardia
- Chest pain
- Rales and crackles
- Increased fremitus
- Egophony
- Dullness on percussion of affected lobes

Medical Treatment

May include the following:

- Prevention via pneumococcal vaccination for children with chronic respiratory illnesses
- Antimicrobial agents
- Supplemental oxygen
- Incentive spirometry
- Hydration
- Arterial blood gas (ABG) assessment

Nursing Diagnoses

May include the following:

- Impaired gas exchange
- Ineffective breathing pattern
- Hyperthermia
- Fluid volume deficit
- Pain
- Anxiety
- Knowledge deficit

Nursing Implications

May include the following:

- Wash hands before and after care
- Encourage prevention via pneumococcal vaccination for children with chronic respiratory illnesses
- Monitor vital signs
- Monitor ABG reports and notify physician of significant change
- Administer antibiotics and monitor for side effects
- Administer prescribed analgesics with attention to respiratory response
- Encourage coughing and deep breathing

Prognosis

Varies depending on cause, age of child, coexisting illnesses, and complications.

Sickle Cell Crisis

Pathophysiology

Sickle cell disease is an autosomal recessive disorder. About 1 in 12 African Americans in the United States carries the gene. Normal hemoglobin is partly or completely replaced by abnormal hemoglobin. Under conditions of dehydration or decreased oxygenation or infection, increased numbers of red blood cells (RBCs) assume irregular shapes (some are sickle shaped). Fragile, sickled cells are poor transporters of oxygen. Sickled cells easily become enmeshed with one another, resulting in early cell destruction, clogging of small blood vessels, and tissue necrosis. "Pain crisis" or vaso-occlusive crisis occurs. Organs such as the liver, spleen, kidneys, and brain may be damaged.

Signs and Symptoms

May include the following:
- Hemoglobin S in blood
- Anorexia
- Increased susceptibility to infection
- Small for age
- Pain—frequently in the abdomen

Common Causes of Hospital Admission

- Infection resulting in increased sickling and resultant pain crisis
- Dehydration resulting in increased sickling and resultant pain crisis
- Cerebral vascular accident (vaso-occlusion of blood vessels in brain)

Medical Treatment

May include the following:
- Supplemental oxygen
- Analgesics
- IV fluids
  - Fluids are encouraged to be at least 1½ times maintenance (see Pediatric Maintenance Fluid Calculation on p 259)
- Prevention: Decrease risk for infection and dehydration to decrease risk for sickling
  - Prophylactic antibiotics may be ordered
  - Supplemental folic acid, B_6, and B_{12} to support RBC production

Nursing Diagnoses

May include the following:

- Pain
- Altered tissue perfusion
- Altered growth and development
- Potential for infection
- Constipation related to analgesic use
- Knowledge deficit

Nursing Implications

- Hand washing before and after care to decrease risk for infection
- Teach child and family the role of infection and hydration in pain crisis prevention
- Encourage fluids to 1½ times usual maintenance amount
- Monitor need for and administer analgesics as needed
- Monitor for and provide ordered medication for analgesic-induced constipation
- Provide emotional support for chronic illness
- Refer to support groups

Seizures

Pathophysiology

A convulsion caused by a sudden discharge of electrical activity in the brain. Generalized seizures are caused by abnormal electrical activity throughout the brain. Partial seizures are caused by abnormal electrical activity in a limited area of the brain.

Common Causes

- Fever
- Increased intracranial pressure from:
  - Hydrocephaly
  - Infection (encephalitis or meningitis)
  - Tumor
  - Head trauma
  - Electrolyte imbalances
  - Hypoglycemia
  - Drug overdose

Signs and Symptoms

Depend on seizure type. Two main types are partial and generalized.

Partial seizures begin in a discreet or "focal" area of the brain	
Simple partial seizure	• No loss of consciousness • Sudden jerking movements may occur, or child may turn head to side or have visual changes • One type of simple partial seizure is the Jacksonian seizure; in the "Jacksonian march," sudden movements begin in one part of the body and progress or "march" to other body parts
Complex partial seizure	• Similar to simple partial but with loss of consciousness • Child may have uncontrollable laughter, paralysis, or sense unusual smells or tastes

Generalized seizures involve large areas of the brain—often both hemispheres	
Grand mal seizure	• A generalized seizure with loss of consciousness, convulsions, and muscle rigidity (tonic-clonic) • Tongue biting and urinary incontinence may occur • Lasts for 1–2 minutes
Absence seizure	• Known as petit mal seizure—brief lapses of consciousness or vacant staring • Lasts for 2–15 seconds
Myoclonic seizure	• Brief jerking movements • Usually occurs in the first 5 years of life

■ Seizure terminology
  ■ **Neonatal seizures:** Symmetrical flexion of the limbs or repeated smacking or chewing movements of the mouth
  ■ **Febrile seizures:** Seizure caused by fever; usually in children younger than 5 years when the seizure threshold is low; more common in boys
  ■ **Atonic:** Loss of muscle tone

- **Clonic:** Repetitive, jerking movement
- **Tonic:** Stiffening and rigidity of muscles
- **Lennox-Gastaut:** Severe form of epilepsy that may be associated with intellectual disability; type of seizure activity varies
- **Status epilepticus:** Continuous seizures that cannot be controlled
- **Post-ictal:** Period following a seizure

Medical Treatment

May include the following:

- Treatment of underlying causes of increased intracranial pressure
- Medications to prevent seizure activity
- Ketogenic diet: A diet high in fat and low in carbohydrates may be recommended (resulting elevated ketones in the blood reduces seizure rate in some children; note that this diet may lead to dehydration, constipation, renal calculi, elevated cholesterol, and slow growth)

Nursing Diagnoses

May include the following:

- Risk for trauma/suffocation
- Impaired social interaction
- Chronic low self-esteem
- Knowledge deficit

Nursing Implications

May include the following:

- Remove sharp objects from environment
- Roll child onto side after seizure activity
- Assess airway and breathing after seizure activity
- Young children with frequent seizures may need to wear a helmet to prevent head injury
- Educate child and family regarding safety
- Do not force objects into mouth during seizure activity

Prognosis

Varies with type of seizure and age of onset.

Foreign Body Airway Obstruction and CPR Initial Response of Health-Care Provider

Alert Infant or Child Who Has Airway Obstruction Due to Foreign Body

Age 1 Year and Older	Infant
If child is coughing do NOT interfere.	If infant is coughing do NOT interfere.
If coughing stops and child is unable to breathe or make a verbal sound, ask "Are you choking?"	If infant stops coughing, is unable to make a vocal sound, or becomes cyanotic, alternate **back slaps and chest thrusts until object is removed or child becomes unresponsive**
If the child nods "yes," has stopped breathing, or becomes cyanotic, stand behind child and perform **abdominal thrusts** (Heimlich maneuver).	
Continue thrusts until the object is forced out or until the child becomes unresponsive.	**Continue** alternating back slaps and chest thrusts until the object is forced out or until the child becomes unresponsive.

Unresponsive Infant or Child With Foreign Body Airway Obstruction

- If infant or child becomes unresponsive, look into the mouth and remove any visible foreign body.
- Do NOT perform blind finger sweeps.
- Begin CPR if foreign body removal is not possible or if foreign body removal does not result in spontaneous respirations.
  - Look into the mouth before each set of respirations and remove any visible object.

First Responder Health-Care Provider Infant CPR—One or Two Rescuers

Wear gloves if feasible.

■ Assess safety of environment before touching infant

■ Assess baby's responsiveness, movement, and respirations; if absent, see next steps. Note that agonal (gasping or abnormal pattern) or gasping breathing is to be treated the same as no breathing

■ Activate emergency services or call 911 (use cell phone if available) or call code or tell bystander to do so. Send someone for automated external defibrillator (AED)

■ Tilt head back (unless there is a head, neck, or back injury) and deliver two rescue breaths, using the amount of air that you can collect in your puffed cheeks and making sure that the infant's chest rises and falls with each breath

■ Assess pulse in brachial artery (mid–upper arm between biceps and triceps) or carotid artery (neck) for no more than 10 seconds

■ If breathing absent or abnormal, provide rescue breathing every 3-5 seconds

■ If no brachial or carotid pulse is found or pulse is below 60 beats per minute or baby meets lack of normal breathing criteria, see next steps

■ Place the infant or child supine (on the back) on a flat, hard surface
  ■ Begin compression/breathing cycles
    • On the lower half of the sternum, between the nipples
    • Two fingers may be used to administer compressions in the infant
    • Administer 30 chest compressions $\frac{1}{3}$ the depth of the full chest of the baby or at least 1.5 inches
    • Use a rate of AT LEAST 100 compressions per minute (or more)
    • Allow chest to recoil after each compression
  ■ Respirations
    • Gently place head in the sniffing position (unless there is neck injury); jaw thrust may be used if neck movement is inadvisable
    • Administer 2 breaths, making the chest rise. Note that rescuer's mouth may cover the baby's nose and mouth or, if an appropriate sized mask is not available, an inverted adult-sized oxygen mask may be used to administer breaths; the smaller part of the mask that usually covers the adult's nose is placed over the baby's chin

- Continue ratio of 30 chest compressions to 2 breaths (30:2) until advanced responders take over or child begins to move—and/or use AED according to device directions as soon as it is available. If AED use does not restore heart rate and breathing, administer 2 more minutes of CPR compressions and breathing, followed by repeat use of AED, repeating cycle until advanced life support providers take over or child begins to move
- If single rescuer is still alone, activate emergency system (if not done) and retrieve and use AED appropriately
- If second rescuer is involved:
  - Chest compression rate to breath ratio is 15:2 (total rate of 100 compressions/minute)
  - If advanced airway has been placed and two rescuers are active, chest compressions are continuous during breaths
  - Two rescuers switch places every 2 minutes—minimize interruptions in compressions to less than 10 seconds; check pulse rate and rhythm while switching rescuer positions
  - Two rescuers—use AED as soon as it is available (analyze rhythm and shock if indicated)
  - If AED use does not restore heart rate and breathing, administer two more minutes of CPR compressions and breathing, followed by repeat use of AED, repeating cycle until advanced life support providers take over or child begins to move.

First Responder Health-Care Provider Child CPR—One or Two Rescuers

- Check for environmental safety before touching patient
- **Assess for responsiveness; if none, activate emergency services as for infant and send for AED**
- **Follow instructions as for infant CPR and AED use with following adaptations for child:**
  - **Compressions**
    - **Compressions may be administered with heel of one hand or second hand on top of first**
    - **At least $\frac{1}{3}$ anteroposterior (AP) check diameter or 2 inches in depth**
    - Continue CPR until advanced responders take over or until the infant or child starts to move

Adapted from *American Heart Association Guidelines for Choking and CPR* (2015).

Apnea Monitor Set Up

Leads

Apnea monitor leads may vary but are generally placed in the following manner:
- White: Top right (at horizontal nipple line)
- Black: Top left (note: Black and white leads should be just to the sides of the nipples and should be parallel)
- Green: Lower right or left (ground lead)
- Red: Lower left (red is sometimes omitted)

Note: If snap-on leads are used, they should be attached to the electrode before lead placement on the chest.

Alarm Settings

- Cardiac alarm is usually set to sound at 15 bpm above and 15 bpm below age-appropriate resting limits (see heart rate for age on p 185)
- Respiratory alarm limit is usually set to sound if there is no respiration for 15 seconds

Children's Fears Related to Hospitalization

Age	Common Fears	Nursing Approaches
5 mo–3 yr	• Separation from mother or usual caregiver • Punishment	• Encourage rooming in • Encourage patient to bring familiar objects from home such as toys or blankets
1–18 yr	• Bodily harm	• Explain procedures in simple terms • Do not inform the child of painful procedures too far in advance • Demonstrate procedures with dolls • Be honest regarding painful procedures • Do not discourage crying • Allow parents to be with child during painful procedures when possible

Continued

Children's Fears Related to Hospitalization—cont'd

Age	Common Fears	Nursing Approaches
6–18 yr	• Separation from parents • Separation from peers • Loss of control	• A school-aged child or adolescent may fear harm that may cause him or her to "look different" (body mutilation) • Encourage visits from family and friends • Encourage use of telephone and e-mail to maintain family and peer contact • Allow choices when possible • Explain procedures in simple terms • Do not discourage crying

Adapted from Holloway, B.W. (2004). Nurse's Fast Facts. F.A. Davis, Philadelphia.

Children's Understanding of Death

Age	Usual Understanding
Birth–1 yr	No concept
1–3 yr	Believes death is temporary and reversible May believe his or her thoughts or actions caused another person's death
4–8 yr	Begins to understand permanence of death May view death as separation May worry about effect of own death on family
8 yr and older	Understands permanence of death May begin to face reality of own mortality

Nursing Approaches With Child and Family Who Face Death

• Allow child and family to ask questions regarding illness and prognosis; be aware that parents often feel responsible for child's condition

Continued

Children's Understanding of Death—cont'd

Nursing Approaches With Child and Family Who Face Death

- Determine child's concept of death and support system before providing answers
- Consider wishes of parents when providing answers
- Allow liberal visiting for siblings and parents; ensure that family has access to support from a minister from their own faith and that religious activities are not hindered

Adapted from Holloway, B. W. (2004). *Nurse's Fast Facts.* Philadelphia, PA: F. A. Davis.

Age-Appropriate Play and Diversional Activities for Hospitalized Children

Age	Appropriate Activity for Child With Nurse, Family, or Other Caregivers
Birth–1 mo	• Cuddle • Rock • Smile at and talk to infant • Place a mobile over bed
2–6 mo	• Provide a nonbreakable mirror at eye level • Provide solid, one-piece toys without detachable parts that do not fit into the mouth and that do not pose a suffocation risk
6–9 mo	• Play peek-a-boo • Provide brightly colored toys that do not fit into the mouth, do not have small detachable parts, and do not pose a suffocation risk • Show pictures in a book
9–12 mo	• Provide blocks and demonstrate stacking • Provide a large ball and demonstrate how to roll the ball • Provide toys and a large container into which toys can be placed and demonstrate placing toys into the container and pouring them out • Play "Where's your nose?" "Where's your mouth?"

Continued

PEDS ACUTE

Age-Appropriate Play and Diversional Activities for Hospitalized Children—cont'd

Age	Appropriate Activity for Child With Nurse, Family, or Other Caregivers
1–3 yr	• Provide pull and push toys (helpful when plan of care includes encouraging ambulation) • Hold a wand filled with commercial "bubble" solution and show the child how to blow bubbles (useful when plan of care includes encouraging deep breathing) • Provide a doll and safe "pretend" hospital supplies such as band aides • Provide a tea set or small pitcher and cup for child to pour and drink (helpful when increased fluid intake is needed) • Read to child
3–6 yr	• Provide simple puzzles • Provide simple board or card games • Provide art supplies • Allow child to use a straw to blow bubbles into a glass (helpful when plan of care includes deep breathing exercises) • Tell the beginning of a story and ask the child to complete the story
School age or adolescent	• Provide books • Provide board games; allow children with noninfectious diseases and noncompromised immune systems to play together • Allow free access to telephone • Allow access to video games if appropriate • Provide art supplies

Adapted from Holloway, B. W. (2004). *Nurse's Fast Facts.* Philadelphia, PA: F. A. Davis.

Encouraging Hospitalized Children to Eat

- Ask about food preferences and communicate these to the dietary department
- If diet allows, give a choice of mealtime beverages
- For toddlers, provide finger foods that can be self-fed
- Unless child expresses a preference, serve food lukewarm rather than hot or cold
- Avoid adding pepper and other spices unless child asks for these; many children dislike spicy food
- Suggest having an "unbirthday" party when meals arrive
- Try to schedule procedures after meals or at least an hour before mealtime
- Allow child to use a tea set or pour liquids from a small pitcher at mealtime
- Encourage family or friends to stay with the child during meals and to eat with the child when possible
- Allow children to eat with other children if possible
- Avoid overemphasizing the need to eat; children who are ill and/or febrile often have decreased appetites and are prone to vomiting

Dosing Safety

Safe dosing for the child is usually based on the following:
- Weight
- Body surface area (calculated using a nomogram that can be found in a pediatric or drug text)
- Age (note that metabolism and excretion of some drugs vary with the age of the child and maturity of the liver and kidneys)

Before administering drug:
- Check the patient's chart for the prescriber's order to determine the following:
  - Name of drug
  - Dose of drug
  - Frequency of dosing
  - Route of administration
  - Check for drug allergies
- Determine why the drug is being given
- Check a drug reference book for special precautions, such as the need to count the heart rate before giving a beta blocker or digoxin
- Determine drug side effects and complications and monitor for both
  - Notify the prescriber if there are signs of serious side effects or complications
- Use a drug reference book to compare the ordered dose to the recommended dose; pounds (lb) must usually be converted to kilograms (kg) to determine safe dosing; to do this:
  - Divide pounds by 2.2 or multiply pounds by 0.45
  - Check approximate accuracy of lb-to-kg conversion by first dividing number of lb by half and then deducting 10% from the answer; for example:
    - Half of 30 lb = 15 lb, subtract 10% (1.5 lb) and the answer is 13.5 kg
    - Note that when 30 lb is divided by 2.2, the answer is 13.6 kg, which is approximately the same answer
  - If the calculated safe dose is significantly different from the ordered dose, then check with prescriber for verification of the dose
    - For children with serious infections, antibiotics are often given in higher doses than recommended in texts; because of potentially serious side effects, sedating or analgesic medication doses should be within the text-stated safe range

- Determine the volume of medication to be given
  - Ask a second person to determine volume (for example, # of mL if medication is liquid) of medication before preparing and giving any medication dose for the first time
- Compare the label on the medication container with the prescriber's order three times:
  1. When taking the medication from storage
  2. Before measuring the medication
  3. After measuring the medication
- Use a syringe (without needle) to measure small doses of liquid PO medications
  - A TB syringe is best for measuring less than 1 mL of liquid medicine
  - When doses are small (less than 0.5 mL), avoid adding extra diluent to the syringe and avoid allowing an air bubble to remain in the syringe because either may cause medication that is in the syringe's dead space (the area in the syringe tip adapter and needle hub) to be administered, thereby increasing the amount of the drug that the child receives

Tips for Administering Oral Medications

For All Children

- Identify the child by checking the name band; do not ask the child if his name is John or Jim, etc.; the child may answer "yes" to any name; do not use the name on the bed for identification; children sometimes change beds while playing
- Allow the parent to give the medication if the child prefers
- Remain in the room until the child has taken all of the medication

For Infants

- Use a syringe to administer small amounts of liquid medications
- If the medication has an unpleasant taste, it can be mixed with a small amount (about 1–5 mL) of juice or syrup
- Medications that have a pleasant taste may be placed into an empty nipple if the infant is able to suck
  - Note: It is acceptable for the nurse to taste a very small amount of liquid medications to determine the taste

- If the infant refuses to suck the medication from a nipple, gently squeeze the infant's cheeks and push a small amount of the liquid medication into the side of the mouth and toward the back of the tongue
- **Do not** place medication on top of the tongue where it may be easily pushed from the mouth
- **Do not** place medication into a bottle with formula or mix it with a feeding because this makes it impossible to know how much medication has been taken if the feeding is not completely consumed
- **Do not** blow into the infant's face to make him swallow; this may cause the infant to gasp and aspirate the liquid into the airway

For Older Children

- Offer choices when possible; for instance, "would you like to take your medication with water or juice?" or ask the child which medication he or she wants to take first
- **Do not** offer a choice; e.g., do not say, "are you ready to take your medicine?" unless taking the medication is optional (such as prn medications); tell the child that it is time to take the medicine
- **Do not** tell a child that medication is candy

Specific Medications

Otic (Ear Drops)

- Identify the child by checking the name band; do not ask the child if his name is John or Jim, etc.; do not use the name on the bed for identification; children sometimes change beds while playing
- Ensure that medication is not cold
- Position the child with the affected ear up
- Straighten the ear canal:
  - For children 3 years of age and younger, gently pull the pinna of the ear down and back
  - For children older than age 3 years, gently pull the pinna of the ear up and back
  - Squeeze the medication onto the side of the outer ear canal; continue to hold the pinna of the ear to keep the ear canal straightened as the liquid runs deeper into the ear

- Avoid dropping medication into the center of the ear canal because this may trap air between the liquid and the tympanic membrane and prevent the medication from coating the entire ear canal
- Continue to hold the pinna of the ear for 1 full minute to allow the medication to reach the tympanic membrane

IM Injections

- Identify the child by checking the name band; do not ask the child if his name is John or Jim, etc.; do not use the name on the bed for identification; children sometimes change beds while playing
- Use a syringe that allows accurate measurement of the proper dose
- Needle gauge should be 23–25
- Length of the needle should be ⅝ inch to 1 inch, depending on size of child and technique used for administration
  - If muscle tissue is stretched and held taut, a ⅝-inch needle may be long enough
  - If muscle tissue is bunched and held between the nurses thumb and fingers, a 1-inch needle is appropriate for all except the smallest of infants
- The maximum amount of medication injected into one site is 1 mL for infants and young children and 2 mL for older children
- When administering IM medications, enter the child's room with someone who is prepared to restrain the child while the injection is being given; do not ask the parent to restrain the child
- Explain the procedure immediately before giving the injection; do not tell a child that an injection will be given until immediately before it is scheduled
- Keep injection materials out of sight until immediately before the injection
- Have assistant restrain child, if necessary; important areas to immobilize are the child's knees, elbows, and area to be injected; avoid contact with the child's mouth to avoid being bitten
- Tell the child that it is okay to cry
- Offer a small decorative bandage for the injection site
- Praise child's efforts to cooperate

Illustrations of IM injection sites follow.

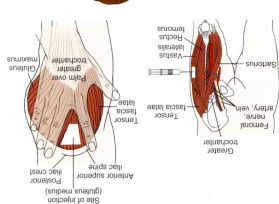

Site of injection
(gluteus medius)

Posterior
iliac crest

Anterior superior
iliac spine

Tensor
fascia latae

Palm over
greater
trochanter

Gluteus
maximus

Tensor fascia latae

Greater
trochanter

Femoral
nerve,
artery, vein

Sartorius

Vastus
lateralis

Rectus
femorus

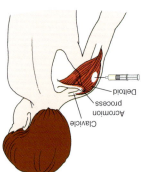

Clavicle

Acromion
process

Deltoid

IV Medications

Preparation for Administration

- Determine the recommended dilution and safe delivery rate for the IV medication to determine method of administration (see following methods)
- Consider the amount of fluid that the child can safely receive (see p 259)
- Consider the compatibility and timing of other IV medications that are ordered
- For the initial IV fluids, potassium (K^+) is added to fluids AFTER the child voids (to ensure that kidneys are functional)

Methods of Administration

- **Heparin locks:** IV medications given through a small port are followed by a "flush" of diluted heparin to prevent clotting of the IV needle or catheter; the amount of flush used depends on the size of the device, but it is usually 1–2 mL; this method can be used when the child does not need IV fluids
- **IV push or bolus:** Medication is pushed into the IV tubing manually or by a pump; this method is useful when immediate effects of the medications are desired or when the IV is running slowly
- **Buretrol:** Medication is added to fluids that are in a calibrated chamber below the IV bag; when using this method, it is important to consider the following:
  - The amount of fluid in the chamber
  - The rate of IV flow
  - The stability of the drug (ampicillin rapidly becomes unstable)
  - The amount of fluid already in the IV tubing
    - Unless the IV is delivering at a rapid rate, the amount of fluid in the chamber (Buretrol) should be small when the medication is added; after the Buretrol is empty, part of the medication will remain in the IV tubing; the amount of fluid needed to clear the line of the medication is equal to the amount of fluid that the tubing will hold—usually 15 to 25 mL
- **Retrograde:** The IV line is clamped while the medication is added to a Y port above the clamp in the IV line; the displaced IV fluid in the line is pushed into a receptacle or empty syringe that is above the injection site and may be discarded; to avoid having any of the medication go into the receptacle or empty syringe, the amount of fluid in the tubing between the medication and the receptacle or syringe must be greater than the volume of the medication being

Starting an IV Line and IV Fluids

- Check the accuracy of all fluid orders with the same care used to calculate drug dosages; remember that infants and young children become dehydrated or fluid-overloaded more rapidly than adults
- Isotonic IV solution for a child younger than 5 years is usually D5.2NS, which is different from adult isotonic solution because of the child's greater extracellular fluid volume
- Isotonic IV solution for a child older than 5 years is usually D5.45NS
- Hang a volume control chamber, such as a Buretrol, below the IV bag
- Use a microdrop device for infants and young children (when using a microdrop device, mL/hr is equal to gtts/min)
- KVO (keep vein open) is a term used when no parenteral fluids are needed but frequent IV medications are being administered; KVO means to set the IV rate to run as slowly as possible without allowing the needle or catheter to develop a clot
- To prevent fluid overload, do not add more than 2 hours' worth of fluid to the Buretrol
- If possible, place the IV tubing on a pump to decrease the possibility of accidental fluid overload
- Arrange assistance to restrain child as described under IM Injections
- Use the smallest needle or IV catheter that will allow delivery of the ordered fluids
- Prepare small sections of tape and any splint that is to be used before inserting the needle or catheter
- Monitor IV site closely for infiltration

injected; this method may be used when IV fluids are running at a slow rate

259

Venous access in child.

Pediatric I.V. Sites

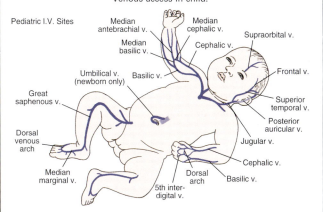

Maintenance Fluids

- Check the accuracy of all fluid orders with the same care used to calculate drug dosages; remember that infants and young children become dehydrated or fluid-overloaded more rapidly than adults
- The following steps can be used to calculate maintenance fluid requirements for children:
  - Note: Maintenance fluids are the amount of PO or IV fluid needed to maintain hydration in a healthy child; additional fluid may be needed to compensate for certain pathological states such as dehydration or sickle cell anemia crisis

Steps in Maintenance Fluid Calculation

1. Convert the child's weight in pounds (lb) to kilograms (kg) by multiplying the number of lb by 0.45
2. Calculate 100 mL of fluid per kg/24 hr for the 1st 10 kg of body wt
3. Calculate 50 mL of fluid per kg/24 hr for the 2nd 10 kg of body wt

4. Calculate 10 to 25 mL of fluid per kg/24 hr for each kg of body wt over 20
5. Add the products of steps 2, 3, and 4 to determine the mL of fluid needed per 24 hours (eliminate any step that is not applicable to the wt of the child)

Note: Add 12% of the total maintenance fluid needed for every degree (Celsius or Centigrade) of body temp over 37.5.

Examples of Maintenance Fluid Calculation for Children

For a 15-Pound Child

- Convert 15 lb to kg by multiplying $15 \times 0.45 = 6.75$ kg
- Allow 100 mL/kg for each of the 6.75 kg = 675 mL
- Divide 675 by 24 (hr) to determine the number of mL fluid/hr = 28
- When using a microdrop device, the rate of IV flow will be the same as mL/hr = 28 gtts/min

For a 70-Pound Child

- Convert 70 lb to kg by multiplying $70 \times 0.45 = 31.5$ kg
- Allow 100 mL/kg for each of the 1st 10 kg = 1000 mL
- Allow 50 mL/kg for each of the 2nd 10 kg = 500 mL
- Allow 20 mL/kg for each of the remaining 11.5 kg = 230 mL
- Note that the physician will determine the exact amount (usually 10–25 mL per kg) for the 3rd and additional kg, based on the child's condition
- Add 1000 mL + 500 mL + 230 mL = 1730 mL
- Divide 1730 by 24 (hr) to determine mL/hr = 72 mL/hr
- The IV rate is 72 gtts/min

Illustration Credits

Pages 73–77 adapted from Mattson, S. (2004). *Core Curriculum for Maternal Newborn Nursing* (3rd ed.). St. Louis: Elsevier.

Page 91 adapted from Murray, S. S. (2002). *Foundations of Maternal-Newborn Nursing* (3rd ed.). St. Louis: Elsevier.

Page 161 from U.S. Department of Agriculture. Discover MyPlate: Nutrition Education for Kindergarten. Retrieved from http://www.fns.usda.gov/discover-myplate-nutrition-education-kindergarten.

Pages 187–194 from the Department of Health and Human Services, National Institutes of Health, National Heart, Lung, and Blood Institute. The Fourth Report on the Diagnosis, Evaluation, and Treatment of High Blood Pressure on Children and Adolescents. Retrieved from https://www.nhlbi.nih.gov/health-pro/guidelines/current/hypertension-pediatric-jnc-4.

Pages 198–201 published by the Centers for Disease Control and Prevention, November 1, 2009. Source: WHO Child Growth Standards. Retrieved from http://www.cdc.gov/growthcharts/who_charts.htm.

Pages 204–205 published May 30, 2000 (modified 11/21/00). Source: Developed by the National Center for Health Statistics in collaboration with the National Center for Chronic Disease Prevention and Health Promotion (2000). Retrieved from http://www.cdc.gov/growthcharts/clinical_charts.htm.

Page 206–207 published May 30, 2000 (modified 10/16/00). Source: Developed by the National Center for Health Statistics in collaboration with the National Center for Chronic Disease Prevention and Health Promotion (2000). Retrieved from http://www.cdc.gov/growthcharts/clinical_charts.htm.

Selected References

Academy of Breastfeeding Medicine (ABM) Protocol Committee. (2011). ABM clinical protocol #8: Human milk storage information for home use for full-term infants. *Breastfeeding Medicine, 5*(3), 127-130.

Agency for Healthcare Research and Quality (AHRQ). (2014). Evidence-based practice center systematic review protocol project title: Management of postpartum hemorrhage. Retrieved from http://www.effectivehealthcare.ahrq.gov/ehc/products/552/1918/hemorrhage-postpartum-protocol-140611.pdf

American Academy of Pediatrics (AAP). (2011). *Neonatal resuscitation* (6th ed.). Washington, DC: Author.

AAP/American Heart Association (AHA). (2015). *Summary AAP/AHA 2015 guidelines for cardiopulmonary resuscitation and emergency cardiovascular care of the neonate.* Retrieved from https://www2.aap.org/nrp/docs/15535_NRP%20Guidelines%20Flyer_English_FINAL.pdf

American Cancer Society. (2014). Breast cancer prevention and early detection. Retrieved from http://www.cancer.org/acs/groups/cid/documents/webcontent/003165-pdf.pdf

American College of Obstetrics and Gynecology (ACOG). (2007). Screening for chromosomal abnormalities. Practice Bulletin No. 77. *Obstetrics and Gynecology, 109,* 217-227.

American College of Obstetrics and Gynecology (ACOG). (2008). Medical management of ectopic pregnancy. Practice Bulletin No. 94. *Obstetrics and Gynecology, 111,* 1479-1485.

American College of Obstetrics and Gynecology (ACOG). (2009). Intrapartum fetal heart rate monitoring: Nomenclature, interpretation, and general management principles. Practice Bulletin No. 70. *Obstetrics and Gynecology, 106,* 192-202.

American College of Obstetrics and Gynecology (ACOG). (2009). Ultrasonography in pregnancy. Practice Bulletin No. 101. *Obstetrics and Gynecology, 113,* 451-461.

American College of Obstetrics and Gynecology (ACOG). (2010). Management of intrapartum fetal heart rate tracings. Practice Bulletin No. 116. *Obstetrics and Gynecology, 106,* 1232-1240.

American College of Obstetrics and Gynecology (ACOG). (2011). Breast cancer screening. Practice Bulletin No. 122. *Obstetrics and Gynecology, 118,* 372-382.

American College of Obstetrics and Gynecology (ACOG). (2012). Noninvasive prenatal testing for fetal aneuploidy. Committee Opinion No. 545. *Obstetrics and Gynecology, 120,* 1532-1534.

American College of Obstetrics and Gynecology (ACOG). (2012). Prediction and prevention of preterm birth. Practice Bulletin No. 130. *Obstetrics and Gynecology, 120,* 964-973.

American College of Obstetrics and Gynecology (ACOG). (2012). Screening for cervical cancer. Practice Bulletin No. 131. *Obstetrics and Gynecology, 120,* 1222-1238.

American College of Obstetrics and Gynecology (ACOG). (2013). Definition of term pregnancy. Committee Opinion No. 579. *Obstetrics and Gynecology, 122,* 1139-1140.

American College of Obstetrics and Gynecology (ACOG). (2013). Gestational diabetes mellitus. Practice Bulletin No. 137. *Obstetrics and Gynecology, 122,* 406-416.

American College of Obstetrics and Gynecology (ACOG). (2013). *Hypertension in pregnancy.* Washington, DC: Author.

American College of Obstetrics and Gynecology (ACOG). (2013). Update on immunizations and pregnancy: Tetanus, diphtheria, and pertussis vaccination. Committee Opinion No. 566. *Obstetrics and Gynecology, 121,* 1411-1414.

American College of Obstetrics and Gynecology (ACOG). (2014). Antepartum fetal surveillance. Practice Bulletin No. 145. *Obstetrics and Gynecology, 120,* 182-192.

American College of Obstetrics and Gynecology (ACOG). (2014). Management of menopausal symptoms. Practice Bulletin No. 141. *Obstetrics and Gynecology, 123,* 202-216.

American College of Obstetrics and Gynecology (ACOG). (2014). Management of preterm labor. Practice Bulletin No. 127. *Obstetrics and Gynecology, 119,* 1308-1317.

American College of Obstetrics and Gynecology (ACOG). (2014). Method for estimating due date. Committee Opinion No. 611. *Obstetrics and Gynecology, 124,* 863-866.

American College of Obstetrics and Gynecology (ACOG). (2015). The Apgar score. Committee Opinion No. 644. *Obstetrics and Gynecology, 126*:e52-55.

American College of Obstetrics and Gynecology (ACOG). (2015). Prenatal and perinatal human immunodeficiency virus testing: Expanded recommendations. Committee Opinion No. 635. *Obstetrics and Gynecology, 125*, 1544-1547.

Association of Women's Health, Obstetric and Neonatal Nurses (AWHONN). (2011). *Nursing care of the woman receiving regional analgesia/anesthesia in labor* (2nd ed.). Washington, DC: Author.

Association of Women's Health, Obstetric and Neonatal Nurses (AWHONN). (2011). *Obstetric hemorrhage.* Washington, DC: Author.

Association of Women's Health, Obstetric and Neonatal Nurses (AWHONN). (2015). Guidelines for oxytocin administration after birth: AWHONN practice brief No. 2. *Journal of Obstetric, Gynecologic, and Neonatal Nursing, 00*, 1-3. DOI: 10.1111/1552-6909.12528

Association of Women's Health, Obstetric and Neonatal Nurses (AWHONN). (2014). Quantification of blood loss: AWHONN practice brief No. 1. *Journal of Obstetric, Gynecologic, and Neonatal Nursing, 00,* 1-3. DOI: 10.1111/1552-6909.12519

Saslow, D., Solomon, D., Lawson, H., Killackey, M., Kulasigsingam, S., Cain, J., et al. (2012). American Cancer Society, American Society for Colposcopy and Cervical Pathology, and American Society for Clinical Pathology screening guidelines for the prevention and early detection of cervical cancer. *Journal of Lower Genital Tract Disease, 16*(3), 1-29.

U.S. Department of Health and Human Services: Division of Women's Health. (2011). *Your guide to breastfeeding.* Washington, DC: Author.

Index

Page numbers followed by "f" denote figures

270